FATTY LIVER DIET COOKBOOK

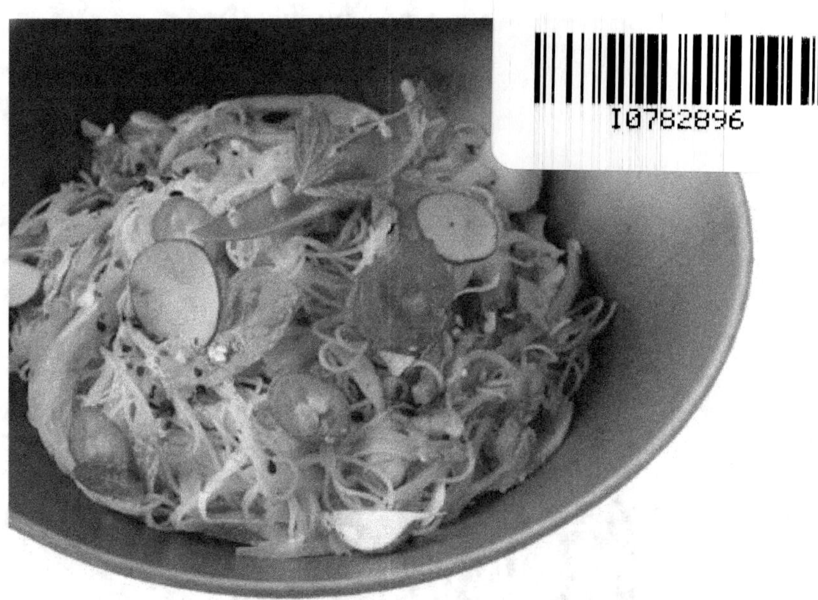

DR. VICKIE STOCK

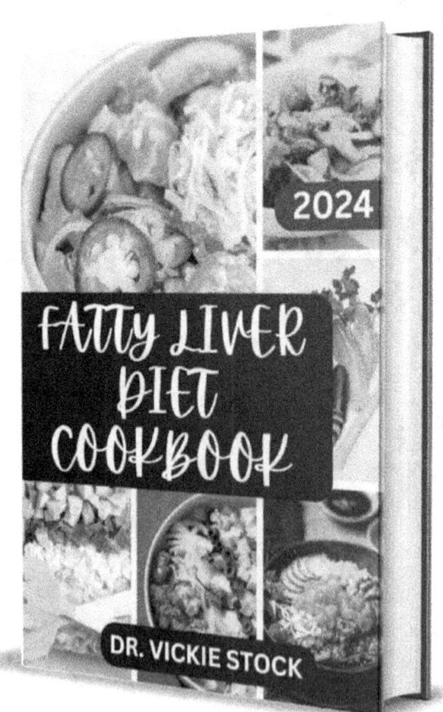
2024
FATTY LIVER
DIET
COOKBOOK
DR. VICKIE STOCK

TABLE OF CONTENT

INTRODUCTION

Fatty liver disease, encompassing non-alcoholic fatty liver disease (NAFLD) and alcoholic fatty liver disease, represents a prevalent and increasingly recognized health concern worldwide.

NAFLD, often linked with sedentary lifestyles and poor dietary habits, is characterized by the accumulation of fat in the liver of individuals who consume minimal or no alcohol. On the other hand, alcoholic fatty liver disease stems from chronic alcohol abuse, leading to liver inflammation and fat deposition.

The global prevalence of NAFLD has surged in parallel with rising rates of obesity, type 2 diabetes, and metabolic syndrome. It is estimated that approximately 25% of the world's population has NAFLD, making it the most common liver disorder.

Moreover, NAFLD can progress to more severe forms of liver disease, including non-alcoholic steatohepatitis (NASH), liver fibrosis, cirrhosis, and hepatocellular carcinoma.

Conversely, alcoholic fatty liver disease remains a leading cause of liver-related morbidity and mortality, particularly in regions where alcohol consumption is prevalent. Chronic alcohol consumption can result in liver damage, inflammation, and ultimately, liver failure if left unchecked.

Understanding the prevalence and implications of fatty liver disease is crucial for public health initiatives, early detection, and effective management strategies to mitigate its impact on individual health and healthcare systems worldwide.

Importance of lifestyle modifications and dietary interventions in managing the condition.

Lifestyle modifications and dietary interventions play a pivotal role in managing fatty liver disease, offering significant potential for improving liver health and preventing disease progression. These interventions are especially crucial given the lack of specific pharmacological treatments for many individuals with fatty liver disease.

By adopting healthier lifestyle habits, such as engaging in regular physical activity and making dietary changes, individuals can effectively address underlying risk factors contributing to the development and progression of the condition.

Lifestyle modifications aim to target key factors implicated in fatty liver disease, including obesity, insulin resistance, and metabolic dysfunction.

Regular exercise promotes weight loss, improves insulin sensitivity, and reduces liver fat accumulation. It also enhances cardiovascular health and overall well-being.

Incorporating a balanced diet rich in fruits, vegetables, whole grains, lean proteins, and healthy fats can help optimize liver function and mitigate inflammation. Furthermore, limiting intake of saturated fats, refined carbohydrates, added sugars, and processed foods helps minimize liver stress and reduce the risk of disease exacerbation.

Lifestyle modifications extend beyond physical activity and diet to encompass stress management, adequate sleep, and abstaining from alcohol consumption for individuals with non-alcoholic fatty liver disease.

By empowering individuals to take control of their health through lifestyle changes, healthcare professionals can facilitate long-term management of fatty liver disease and improve health outcomes for affected individuals.

Below is the Picture of a damaged Liver

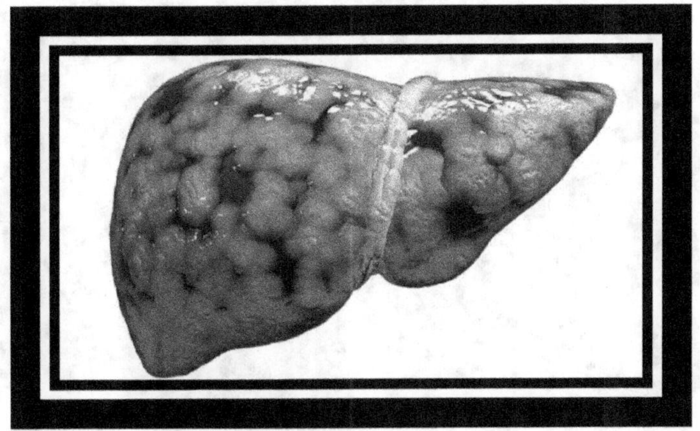

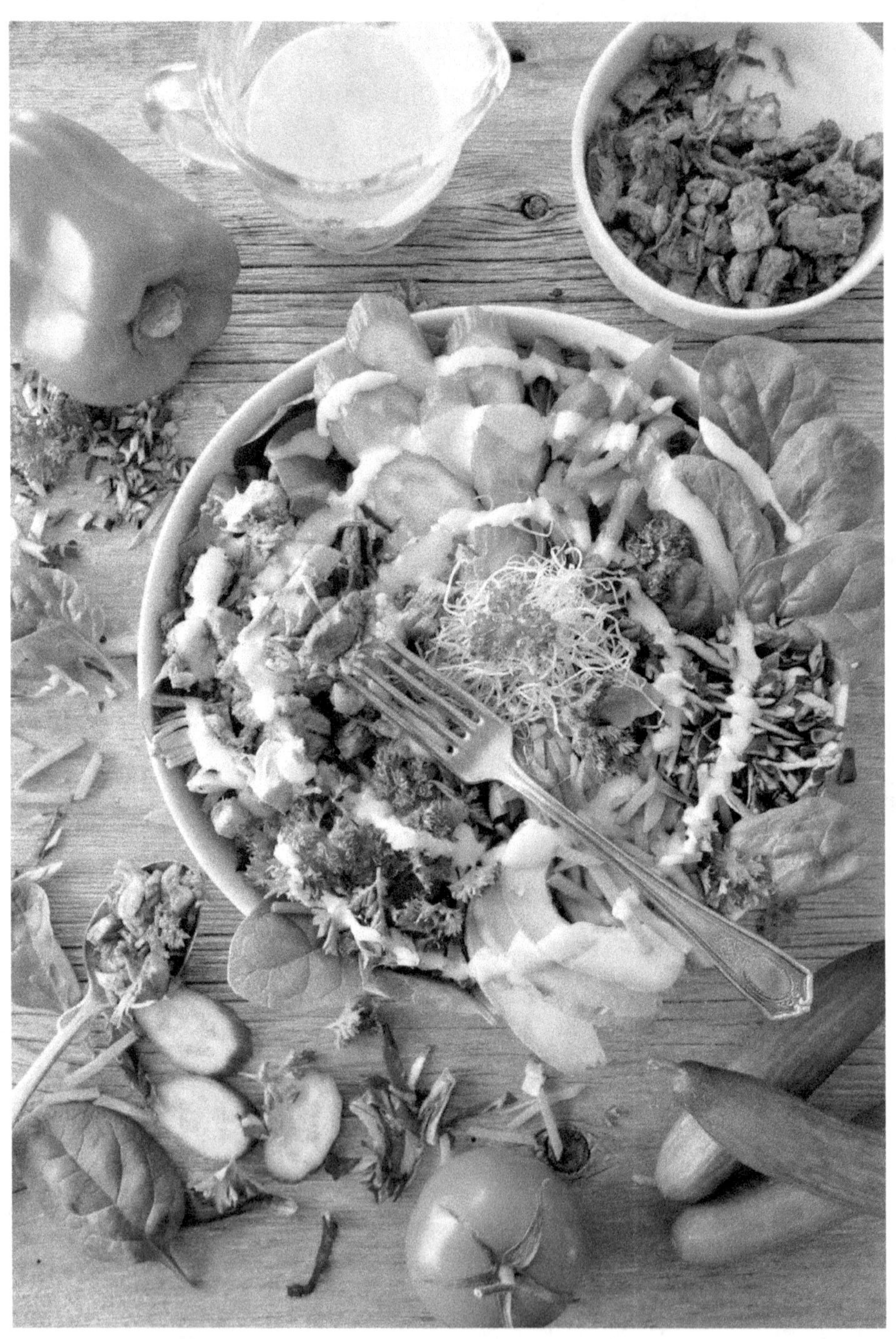

CHAPTER ONE: What is Fatty Liver Disease?

Fatty liver disease encompasses a spectrum of conditions characterized by the accumulation of fat in the liver cells, leading to impaired liver function. The two primary types of fatty liver disease are non-alcoholic fatty liver disease (NAFLD) and alcoholic fatty liver disease.

NAFLD is the most common form of fatty liver disease and occurs in individuals who do not consume excessive amounts of alcohol. It is closely associated with obesity, insulin resistance, type 2 diabetes, high cholesterol, and metabolic syndrome.

NAFLD can range from simple steatosis, characterized by excess fat accumulation in the liver, to non-alcoholic steatohepatitis (NASH), which involves liver inflammation and damage. If left untreated, NASH can progress to more severe liver conditions, such as fibrosis, cirrhosis, and even liver cancer.

Alcoholic fatty liver disease, on the other hand, develops due to excessive alcohol consumption over time. The toxic effects of alcohol lead to fat accumulation in the liver cells, causing inflammation and liver damage.

Alcoholic fatty liver disease can progress from simple fatty liver to more severe conditions, including alcoholic hepatitis and cirrhosis, which are associated with significant morbidity and mortality. Effective management of both NAFLD and alcoholic fatty liver disease involves lifestyle modifications, such as dietary changes, weight loss, and alcohol cessation, along with close monitoring by healthcare professionals to prevent disease progression and complications.

Risk factors and common causes.

Fatty liver disease arises from a combination of genetic, environmental, and lifestyle factors. Understanding its risk factors and common causes is crucial for prevention and effective management.

Obesity and Metabolic Syndrome: Excess body weight, particularly abdominal obesity, is a significant risk factor for fatty liver disease. Metabolic syndrome, characterized by a combination of obesity, insulin resistance, high blood pressure, and abnormal lipid levels, increases the likelihood of developing NAFLD.

Insulin Resistance and Type 2 Diabetes: Insulin resistance, a condition in which cells become less responsive to insulin, is closely linked to fatty liver disease. Individuals with insulin resistance are at higher risk of developing NAFLD, particularly if they have type 2 diabetes.

High Cholesterol and Triglycerides: Elevated levels of cholesterol and triglycerides in the blood contribute to the accumulation of fat in the liver, increasing the risk of NAFLD and its progression to more severe forms.

Poor Dietary Habits: Diets high in saturated fats, refined carbohydrates, and added sugars can promote fat deposition in the liver, exacerbating fatty liver disease. Excessive calorie intake, particularly from sugary beverages and processed foods, contributes to liver fat accumulation.

Alcohol Consumption: Excessive alcohol consumption is a well-established cause of alcoholic fatty liver disease. Chronic alcohol abuse leads to liver inflammation, oxidative stress, and fat accumulation, predisposing individuals to liver damage and disease progression.

Medications and Toxins: Certain medications, such as corticosteroids, tamoxifen, and methotrexate, can cause or exacerbate fatty liver disease. Additionally, exposure to environmental toxins and pollutants may contribute to liver damage and fat accumulation.

Genetic Factors: Genetic predisposition plays a role in the development of fatty liver disease. Some individuals may have genetic variants that increase their susceptibility to liver fat accumulation and disease progression.

By addressing these risk factors through lifestyle modifications, such as adopting a healthy diet, maintaining a healthy weight, exercising regularly, limiting alcohol intake, and avoiding harmful medications and toxins, individuals can reduce their risk of developing fatty liver disease and improve their liver health. Regular monitoring and screening for risk factors are essential for early detection and intervention.

Symptoms and complications associated with the condition.

Fatty liver disease often progresses silently in its early stages, with many individuals experiencing few or no noticeable symptoms. However, as the condition advances, symptoms may develop, and complications can arise, posing significant health risks.

➤ **Symptoms:**

Fatigue: Persistent tiredness and lack of energy are common symptoms of fatty liver disease, often attributed to impaired liver function and inflammation.

Abdominal Discomfort: Some individuals may experience discomfort or pain in the upper right abdomen, where the liver is located. This discomfort may be dull or sharp and can worsen after eating fatty or heavy meals.

Weight Loss or Appetite Changes: Unintended weight loss or changes in appetite may occur in some individuals with advanced fatty liver disease, particularly in cases of liver inflammation or cirrhosis.

Weakness and Malaise: Feelings of weakness, malaise, or a general sense of unwellness may accompany fatty liver disease, reflecting the systemic impact of liver dysfunction on overall health.

➢ **Complications:**

Liver Inflammation (Non-alcoholic Steatohepatitis, NASH): Inflammation of the liver, known as NASH, is a severe form of fatty liver disease characterized by liver cell damage and inflammation. NASH can progress to fibrosis, cirrhosis, and liver failure if left untreated.

Liver Fibrosis and Cirrhosis: Prolonged inflammation and scarring of the liver tissue can lead to fibrosis, where healthy liver tissue is replaced by scar tissue. Over time, extensive fibrosis can progress to cirrhosis, a severe and irreversible condition characterized by widespread scarring and impaired liver function.

Liver Failure: Advanced fatty liver disease, particularly cirrhosis, increases the risk of liver failure, where the liver loses its ability to function adequately, leading to life-threatening complications such as hepatic encephalopathy and ascites.

Liver Cancer (Hepatocellular Carcinoma): Individuals with fatty liver disease, especially those with advanced fibrosis or cirrhosis, are at increased risk of developing hepatocellular carcinoma, a type of liver cancer with poor prognosis if not detected and treated early.

Recognizing the symptoms and complications of fatty liver disease is essential for timely diagnosis and intervention. Early detection and management through lifestyle modifications, medical treatment, and regular monitoring can help prevent disease progression and improve outcomes for individuals with fatty liver disease.

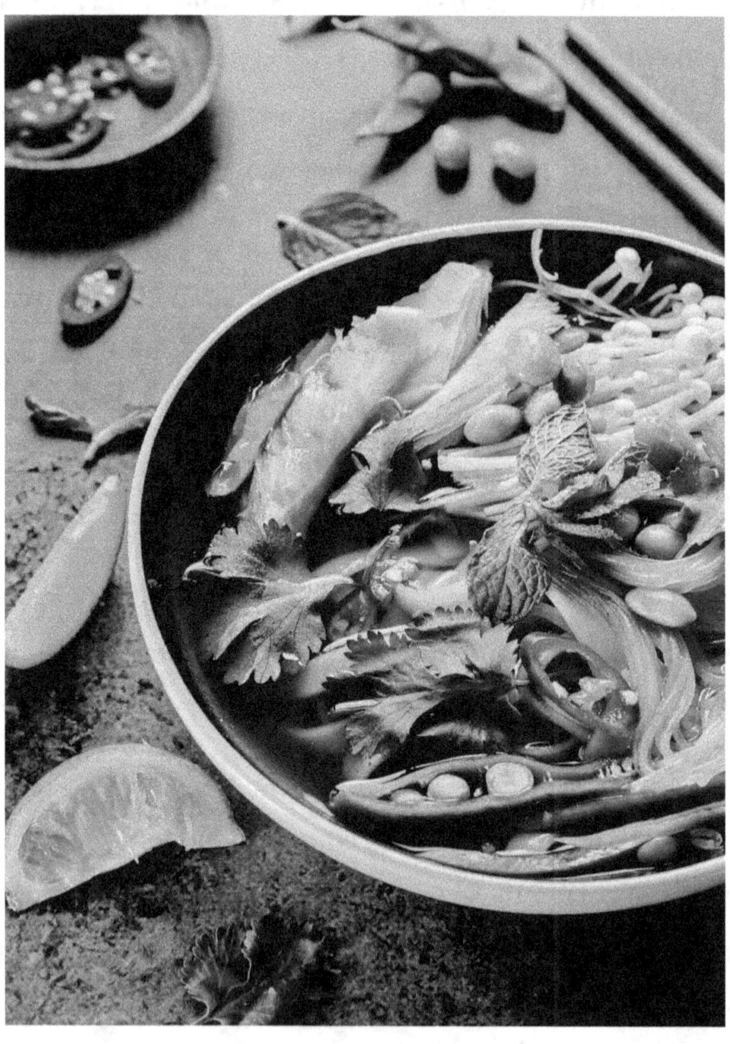

CHAPTER TWO: The Fatty Liver Diet: Eating for Liver Health

Principles of a liver-friendly diet.

A liver-friendly diet is a cornerstone in managing fatty liver disease and promoting overall liver health. The principles of a liver-friendly diet revolve around making nutritious food choices that support liver function, reduce inflammation, and minimize fat accumulation in the liver. Key components of a liver-friendly diet include:

Firstly, emphasizing whole, unprocessed foods such as fruits, vegetables, whole grains, and legumes. These foods are rich in vitamins, minerals, antioxidants, and fiber, which help protect liver cells from damage and aid in digestion and detoxification processes.

Secondly, incorporating lean sources of protein, such as poultry, fish, tofu, and legumes, while limiting intake of red meat and processed meats. Protein is essential for tissue repair and supports liver function without adding excess fat to the diet.

Thirdly, choosing healthy fats from sources like avocados, nuts, seeds, and olive oil. These fats provide essential fatty acids that support cellular function and reduce inflammation in the liver.

Additionally, reducing intake of saturated fats, trans fats, and cholesterol, commonly found in fried foods, processed snacks, and fatty meats, helps prevent further liver damage and supports cardiovascular health.

Lastly, staying hydrated by drinking plenty of water throughout the day is crucial for optimal liver function and detoxification.

By following these principles, individuals can help manage fatty liver disease and support overall liver health.

Foods to include: fruits, vegetables, whole grains, lean proteins, healthy fats.

Incorporating a variety of nutrient-rich foods into one's diet is essential for supporting liver health and managing conditions like fatty liver disease. Fruits, vegetables, whole grains, lean proteins, and healthy fats are foundational components of a balanced diet that can provide numerous benefits for liver function and overall well-being.

Fruits and vegetables are rich in vitamins, minerals, antioxidants, and dietary fiber. They help to reduce inflammation, promote liver detoxification, and support digestive health. Colorful options such as berries, leafy greens, citrus fruits, and cruciferous vegetables like broccoli and Brussels sprouts are particularly beneficial.

Whole grains such as brown rice, quinoa, oats, and whole wheat contain fiber, B vitamins, and minerals that support energy production and help regulate blood sugar levels.

These grains provide sustained energy and can help prevent spikes in blood sugar, which is important for individuals with fatty liver disease.

Lean proteins, including poultry, fish, tofu, legumes, and low-fat dairy products, are vital for tissue repair and muscle maintenance. They provide essential amino acids without adding excess saturated fat or cholesterol to the diet. Consuming lean proteins also helps promote satiety and can support weight management, which is crucial for individuals with fatty liver disease.

Healthy fats from sources like avocados, nuts, seeds, and olive oil provide essential fatty acids, such as omega-3 and omega-6, that support cellular function and reduce inflammation. These fats can help improve cholesterol levels and reduce the risk of heart disease, which is often associated with fatty liver disease

By including a variety of these nutrient-dense foods in their diet, individuals can support liver health, manage fatty liver disease, and promote overall well-being.

Foods to limit or avoid: saturated fats, refined carbohydrates, added sugars, processed foods.

Limiting or avoiding certain types of foods is crucial for managing fatty liver disease and promoting liver health. Saturated fats, refined carbohydrates, added sugars, and processed foods are among the main culprits that can contribute to liver inflammation, fat accumulation, and metabolic disturbances.

Saturated fats, found in foods like red meat, full-fat dairy products, and processed meats, can raise levels of LDL cholesterol and promote inflammation in the liver. It's important to minimize intake of these fats and opt for healthier sources of fat, such as unsaturated fats from nuts, seeds, avocados, and olive oil.

Refined carbohydrates, including white bread, white rice, sugary cereals, and pastries, are quickly broken down into sugar in the body, leading to spikes in blood sugar levels and insulin resistance. High intake of refined carbohydrates can contribute to fatty liver disease and metabolic syndrome. Instead, focus on whole grains like brown rice, quinoa, and oats, which provide fiber and nutrients without causing rapid fluctuations in blood sugar.

Added sugars, commonly found in sugary beverages, desserts, candy, and processed foods, can contribute to liver fat accumulation and insulin resistance. Minimizing intake of added sugars is essential for managing fatty liver disease and supporting overall health.

Processed foods, such as fast food, packaged snacks, and convenience meals, often contain high amounts of unhealthy fats, refined carbohydrates, added sugars, and additives. These foods offer little nutritional value and can contribute to weight gain, inflammation, and liver damage.

CHAPTER THREE: Lifestyle strategies for Managing fatty Liver Disease

Importance of regular physical activity and exercise.

Regular physical activity and exercise play a crucial role in managing fatty liver disease and promoting overall liver health. Engaging in regular exercise offers numerous benefits that can help individuals with fatty liver disease improve their condition and reduce the risk of complications.

Exercise helps to promote weight loss and reduce excess fat accumulation in the liver, which is essential for improving liver function and reducing inflammation.

Additionally, physical activity helps to improve insulin sensitivity, which can help individuals with fatty liver disease better regulate their blood sugar levels and reduce the risk of developing type 2 diabetes.

Exercise has been shown to reduce levels of triglycerides and cholesterol in the blood, which are risk factors for fatty liver disease and cardiovascular disease.

By improving lipid profiles, exercise can help individuals with fatty liver disease lower their risk of heart disease and other related conditions. Furthermore, regular physical activity has been associated with improvements in overall fitness, energy levels, and mood, which can contribute to better quality of life for individuals living with fatty liver disease. Overall, incorporating regular exercise into a comprehensive treatment plan can have significant benefits for individuals with fatty liver disease, supporting liver health and overall well-being.

Tips for incorporating exercise into daily routine.

Incorporating exercise into one's daily routine is essential for individuals managing fatty liver disease. However, finding the time and motivation to exercise regularly can be challenging. Here are some practical tips to help individuals incorporate exercise into their daily lives:

Set Realistic Goals: Start by setting achievable exercise goals that align with your fitness level and schedule. Whether it's aiming for a certain number of steps per day or committing to a specific workout routine, setting realistic goals can help you stay motivated and track your progress.

Find Activities You Enjoy: Choose activities that you genuinely enjoy, whether it's walking, cycling, swimming, dancing, or gardening. When exercise feels like fun rather than a chore, you're more likely to stick with it long term.

Schedule Exercise Sessions: Treat exercise like any other appointment by scheduling it into your daily or weekly calendar.

Set aside dedicated time for physical activity, whether it's in the morning before work, during your lunch break, or in the evening after dinner.

Be Flexible: Life can be unpredictable, so be willing to adapt your exercise routine to accommodate changes in your schedule. If you miss a workout, don't dwell on it—simply reschedule it for another time or find alternative ways to stay active.

Incorporate Exercise into Daily Activities: Look for opportunities to sneak in extra physical activity throughout the day. Take the stairs instead of the elevator, walk or cycle instead of driving for short trips, and engage in active hobbies or household chores.

Make it Social: Exercise with friends, family members, or a workout buddy to make it more enjoyable and hold each other accountable. Joining group fitness classes or sports teams can also provide social support and motivation.

Reward Yourself: Celebrate your exercise accomplishments by rewarding yourself with non-food rewards, such as buying new workout gear, treating yourself to a massage, or enjoying a relaxing bath.

By implementing these tips, individuals can make exercise a sustainable and enjoyable part of their daily routine, ultimately supporting their efforts to manage fatty liver disease and improve overall health.

Stress management techniques and their impact on liver health.

Stress management techniques are crucial for individuals with fatty liver disease as chronic stress can exacerbate liver inflammation and contribute to disease progression. Implementing effective stress management strategies not only improves mental well-being but also positively impacts liver health. Here are some techniques and their potential benefits:

Mindfulness Meditation: Mindfulness meditation involves focusing on the present moment without judgment, which can help reduce stress levels and promote relaxation. Research suggests that regular meditation practice may lower inflammation markers in the body, including those related to liver health.

Deep Breathing Exercises: Deep breathing exercises, such as diaphragmatic breathing or progressive muscle relaxation, activate the body's relaxation response and reduce the physiological symptoms of stress. By promoting relaxation, deep breathing techniques can help alleviate stress-related liver inflammation.

Yoga and Tai Chi: Practices like yoga and tai chi combine physical movement with breath awareness and meditation, making them effective tools for stress reduction. These mind-body exercises have been shown to decrease stress hormones, improve mood, and enhance overall well-being, which can benefit liver health.

Regular Exercise: Engaging in regular physical activity is not only beneficial for liver health but also an effective stress management tool. Exercise releases endorphins, natural mood-boosting chemicals in the brain, and reduces levels of stress hormones like cortisol.

Healthy Lifestyle Habits: Maintaining a balanced diet, getting adequate sleep, and limiting caffeine and alcohol intake are essential lifestyle habits that can help manage stress and support liver health.

By incorporating these stress management techniques into their daily routine, individuals with fatty liver disease can better cope with stressors, reduce liver inflammation, and improve overall liver health. It's important to find the techniques that work best for each individual and to prioritize self-care in managing this chronic condition.

7-Day Fatty Liver-Friendly Meal Plan

Day 1

> Breakfast: Oatmeal with Strawberries and Walnuts

Instructions: Cook oatmeal according to package instructions. Top with fresh sliced strawberries and chopped walnuts.

> Lunch: Spinach and Quinoa Salad with Avocado and Black Beans

Instructions: Cook quinoa according to package instructions. In a bowl, combine cooked quinoa with fresh spinach, diced avocado, and drained black beans. Drizzle with olive oil and toss gently to coat.

> Dinner: Baked Salmon with Broccoli and Brown Rice

Instructions: Preheat oven to 375°F (190°C). Place salmon fillets on a baking sheet lined with parchment paper. Season with salt, pepper, and your favorite herbs. Bake for 15-20 minutes or until salmon is cooked through. Steam broccoli until tender. Serve salmon with steamed broccoli and cooked brown rice.

Day 2

> Breakfast: Greek Yogurt Parfait with Blueberries and Almonds

Instructions: In a bowl or glass, layer Greek yogurt with fresh blueberries, sliced almonds, and chia seeds.

> Lunch: Kale and Quinoa Bowl with Roasted Sweet Potatoes and Kidney Beans

Instructions: Roast sweet potato cubes in the oven at 400°F (200°C) for 20-25 minutes or until tender.

In a bowl, combine cooked quinoa, chopped kale, roasted sweet potatoes, and drained kidney beans. Drizzle with olive oil and season with salt and pepper to taste.

> ➤ Dinner: Stir-fried Tofu with Mixed Vegetables and Brown Rice

Instructions: Heat oil in a pan over medium heat. Add diced tofu and stir-fry until golden brown. Add chopped mixed vegetables (such as bell peppers, broccoli, and carrots) and cook until tender. Serve stir-fried tofu and vegetables with cooked brown rice.

Day 3

> ➤ Breakfast: Whole Grain Toast with Mashed Avocado and Sliced Tomatoes

Instructions: Toast whole grain bread until golden brown. Mash avocado and spread it on the toast. Top with sliced tomatoes and a sprinkle of salt and pepper.

> ➤ Lunch: Beet and Spinach Salad with Walnuts and Balsamic Vinaigrette

Instructions: In a bowl, combine fresh spinach leaves, thinly sliced beets, chopped walnuts, and shredded carrots. Drizzle with balsamic vinaigrette and toss to coat.

➢ Dinner: Grilled Chicken Breast with Quinoa Pilaf and Steamed Green Beans

Instructions: Season chicken breast with salt, pepper, and your favorite herbs. Grill until cooked through. Serve with cooked quinoa pilaf (cooked quinoa mixed with sautéed onions, garlic, and diced vegetables) and steamed green beans.

Day 4

➢ Breakfast: Kale Berry Smoothie with Banana and Chia Seeds

Instructions: Blend kale, mixed berries, banana, and chia seeds with your choice of liquid (water, almond milk, or coconut water) until smooth.

➢ Lunch: Lentil Soup with Carrots, Celery, and Garlic

Instructions: In a large pot, sauté chopped onions, garlic, carrots, and celery until softened. Add dried lentils and vegetable broth. Simmer until lentils are tender. Season with salt, pepper, and herbs.

➢ Dinner: Baked Sweet Potatoes Stuffed with Black Beans, Salsa, and Avocado

Instructions: Preheat oven to 400°F (200°C). Bake sweet potatoes until tender. Split open and fill with warmed black beans, salsa, and sliced avocado.

> ➢ Breakfast: Chia Seed Pudding with Sliced Apples and Cinnamon

Instructions: Mix chia seeds with almond milk in a jar and let it sit in the refrigerator overnight. In the morning, layer the chia seed pudding with sliced apples and a sprinkle of cinnamon.

> ➢ Lunch: Quinoa and Black Bean Salad with Tomatoes and Bell Peppers

Instructions: Cook quinoa according to package instructions. In a bowl, combine cooked quinoa, drained black beans, diced tomatoes, diced bell peppers, and a squeeze of lime juice. Toss gently to combine.

> ➢ Dinner: Grilled Salmon with Roasted Brussels Sprouts and Quinoa

Instructions: Grill salmon fillets until cooked through. Roast Brussels sprouts in the oven at 400°F (200°C) with olive oil, salt, and pepper until golden brown and crispy. Serve with cooked quinoa.

Day 6

> ➢ Breakfast: Overnight Oats with Sliced Strawberries and Chopped Almonds

Instructions: Mix rolled oats with almond milk in a jar and refrigerate overnight. In the morning, top the overnight oats with sliced strawberries and chopped almonds.

> ➢ Lunch: Spinach and Chickpea Salad with Avocado and Lemon-Tahini Dressing

Instructions: In a bowl, combine fresh spinach leaves, drained chickpeas, diced avocado, and a drizzle of lemon-tahini dressing.

➢ Dinner: Vegetable Stir-Fry with Tofu and Brown Rice

Instructions: Stir-fry diced tofu with mixed vegetables (such as bell peppers, broccoli, and snap peas) in a pan with sesame oil and soy sauce. Serve with cooked brown rice.

Day 7

➢ Breakfast: Whole Grain Pancakes with Blueberries and Maple Syrup

Instructions: Prepare whole grain pancake batter according to package instructions. Cook pancakes on a griddle until golden brown. Top with fresh blueberries and a drizzle of maple syrup.

➢ Lunch: Greek Salad with Mixed Greens, Olives, Tomatoes, Cucumber, and Feta Cheese

Instructions: Toss mixed greens with halved cherry tomatoes, sliced cucumber, Kalamata olives, and crumbled feta cheese. Drizzle with olive oil and red wine vinegar.

➢ Dinner: Baked Chicken Thighs with Roasted Carrots and Quinoa

Instructions: Season chicken thighs with salt, pepper, and herbs. Bake in the oven at 375°F (190°C) until cooked through. Serve with roasted carrots and cooked quinoa.

CHAPTER FOUR: Fatty Liver Breakfast Recipes

1: Avocado and Spinach Breakfast Wrap

Ingredients:

- 1 whole grain tortilla
- 1/2 ripe avocado, mashed
- 1/4 cup cooked quinoa
- 1/4 cup baby spinach leaves
- 2 eggs, scrambled
- Salt and pepper to taste

Instructions:

1. Heat the whole grain tortilla in a skillet until warm.
2. Spread the mashed avocado evenly over the tortilla.
3. Layer the cooked quinoa, baby spinach leaves, and scrambled eggs on top of the avocado.
4. Season with salt and pepper to taste.
5. Roll up the tortilla to form a wrap.
6. Slice the wrap in half and serve immediately.

Nutritional Value (per serving):

- Calories: 350
- Protein: 16g

- ➤ Carbohydrates: 26g
- ➤ Fat: 21g
- ➤ Fiber: 8g

Servings: 1

Difficulty: Easy

Preparation Time: 10 minutes

2: Berry Chia Seed Pudding

Ingredients:

- ➤ 1/4 cup chia seeds
- ➤ 1 cup unsweetened almond milk
- ➤ 1/2 teaspoon vanilla extract
- ➤ 1/2 cup mixed berries (such as strawberries, blueberries, and raspberries)
- ➤ 1 tablespoon chopped almonds
- ➤ 1 teaspoon honey or maple syrup (optional)

Instructions:

1. In a bowl, mix together chia seeds, almond milk, and vanilla extract. Stir well to combine.
2. Let the mixture sit for at least 30 minutes or refrigerate overnight, stirring occasionally until it thickens into a pudding-like consistency.

3. Once the chia pudding has thickened, layer it with mixed berries in a serving glass or bowl.

4. Top with chopped almonds and drizzle with honey or maple syrup if desired.

5. Serve chilled.

Nutritional Value (per serving):

➢ Calories: 250

➢ Protein: 8g

➢ Carbohydrates: 25g

➢ Fat: 14g

➢ Fiber: 13g

Servings: 1

Difficulty: Easy

Preparation Time: 5 minutes (plus chilling time)

3: Green Smoothie Bowl

Ingredients:

➢ 1 ripe banana, frozen

➢ 1 cup baby spinach leaves

➢ 1/2 cup chopped kale leaves, stems removed

➢ 1/4 cup unsweetened almond milk

➢ 1 tablespoon almond butter

- ➤ 1 tablespoon chia seeds
- ➤ Toppings: sliced strawberries, blueberries, granola, and shredded coconut

Instructions:

1. In a blender, combine the frozen banana, baby spinach, chopped kale, almond milk, almond butter, and chia seeds.
2. Blend until smooth and creamy, adding more almond milk if needed to reach desired consistency.
3. Pour the smoothie into a bowl.
4. Top with sliced strawberries, blueberries, granola, and shredded coconut.
5. Serve immediately and enjoy with a spoon!

Nutritional Value (per serving):

- ➤ Calories: 350
- ➤ Protein: 8g
- ➤ Carbohydrates: 45g
- ➤ Fat: 17g
- ➤ Fiber: 12g

Servings: 1

Difficulty: Easy

Preparation Time: 5 minutes

4: Veggie Egg Muffins

Ingredients:

- ➢ 4 large eggs
- ➢ 1/4 cup diced bell peppers (any color)
- ➢ 1/4 cup diced tomatoes
- ➢ 1/4 cup diced mushrooms
- ➢ 1/4 cup chopped spinach leaves
- ➢ Salt and pepper to taste
- ➢ Cooking spray or olive oil for greasing

Instructions:

1. Preheat the oven to 350°F (175°C). Grease a muffin tin with cooking spray or olive oil.
2. In a bowl, whisk together the eggs until well beaten. Season with salt and pepper.
3. Divide the diced bell peppers, tomatoes, mushrooms, and chopped spinach evenly among the muffin cups.
4. Pour the beaten eggs over the vegetables in each muffin cup, filling them about 3/4 full.
5. Bake in the preheated oven for 20-25 minutes or until the egg muffins are set and lightly golden on top.
6. Allow the egg muffins to cool slightly before removing them from the muffin tin.
7. Serve warm or at room temperature.

Nutritional Value (per serving - 2 egg muffins):

- ➢ Calories: 200
- ➢ Protein: 14g
- ➢ Carbohydrates: 5g
- ➢ Fat: 13g
- ➢ Fiber: 2g

Servings: 1 (2 egg muffins)

Difficulty: Easy

Preparation Time: 30 minutes

5: Turmeric Scrambled Tofu

Ingredients:

- ➢ 1/2 block firm tofu, crumbled
- ➢ 1/4 teaspoon ground turmeric
- ➢ 1/4 teaspoon ground cumin
- ➢ 1/4 teaspoon paprika
- ➢ Salt and pepper to taste
- ➢ 1 tablespoon olive oil
- ➢ 1/4 cup diced bell peppers
- ➢ 1/4 cup diced onions
- ➢ 1/4 cup chopped fresh parsley

Instructions:

1. Heat olive oil in a skillet over medium heat. Add diced bell peppers and onions, and sauté until softened.
2. Add crumbled tofu to the skillet and sprinkle with ground turmeric, ground cumin, paprika, salt, and pepper. Cook for 5-7 minutes, stirring occasionally.
3. Once the tofu is heated through and lightly browned, remove from heat and stir in chopped fresh parsley.
4. Serve hot as a delicious and nutritious alternative to scrambled eggs.

Nutritional Value (per serving):

➢ Calories: 180
➢ Protein: 10g
➢ Carbohydrates: 5g
➢ Fat: 14g
➢ Fiber: 2g

Servings: 1

Difficulty: Easy

Preparation Time: 15 minutes

Ingredients:

- 1 small sweet potato, peeled and diced
- 1/4 cup diced red bell pepper
- 1/4 cup diced green bell pepper
- 1/4 cup diced onion
- 1 tablespoon olive oil
- 1/2 teaspoon smoked paprika
- Salt and pepper to taste
- 2 eggs
- Chopped fresh cilantro for garnish (optional)

Instructions:

1. Heat olive oil in a skillet over medium heat. Add diced sweet potato, red bell pepper, green bell pepper, and onion to the skillet.
2. Sprinkle with smoked paprika, salt, and pepper. Cook, stirring occasionally, until sweet potatoes are tender and lightly browned, about 10-12 minutes.
3. Meanwhile, fry eggs to desired doneness in a separate skillet.
4. Once the sweet potato hash is cooked, divide it between serving plates. Top each portion with a fried egg.
5. Garnish with chopped fresh cilantro if desired, and serve hot.

Nutritional Value (per serving):

> Calories: 300

> Protein: 10g

> Carbohydrates: 25g

> Fat: 18g

> Fiber: 4g

Servings: 1

Difficulty: Easy

Preparation Time: 20 minutes

7: Veggie and Egg Breakfast Burrito

Ingredients:

> 1 whole grain tortilla

> 2 eggs, scrambled

> 1/4 cup diced bell peppers (any color)

> 1/4 cup diced tomatoes

> 1/4 cup chopped spinach leaves

> 2 tablespoons shredded low-fat cheese

> Salt and pepper to taste

> Cooking spray or olive oil for greasing

Instructions:

> Heat a skillet over medium heat and lightly coat with cooking spray or olive oil.
> Add diced bell peppers and cook until softened, about 2-3 minutes.
> Add diced tomatoes and chopped spinach leaves to the skillet and cook for an additional 1-2 minutes.
> Push the vegetables to one side of the skillet and add the scrambled eggs to the other side. Cook until eggs are scrambled and fully cooked.
> Warm the whole grain tortilla in the microwave for 10-15 seconds or on a dry skillet for a few seconds on each side.
> Place the scrambled eggs and vegetable mixture onto the tortilla, sprinkle with shredded cheese, and season with salt and pepper.
> Roll up the tortilla to form a burrito and serve immediately.

Nutritional Value (per serving):

> Calories: 300
> Protein: 17g
> Carbohydrates: 24g
> Fat: 14g
> Fiber: 5g

Servings: 1

Difficulty: Easy

Preparation Time: 15 minutes

8: Apple Cinnamon Overnight Oats

Ingredients:

- ➤ 1/2 cup rolled oats
- ➤ 1/2 cup unsweetened almond milk
- ➤ 1/2 medium apple, diced
- ➤ 1 tablespoon chopped walnuts
- ➤ 1/2 teaspoon ground cinnamon
- ➤ 1 teaspoon honey or maple syrup (optional)

Instructions:

1. In a mason jar or airtight container, combine rolled oats, unsweetened almond milk, diced apple, chopped walnuts, ground cinnamon, and honey or maple syrup if using.
2. Stir well to combine all ingredients.
3. Cover the jar or container and refrigerate overnight or for at least 4 hours.
4. In the morning, give the overnight oats a good stir and add more almond milk if desired for a creamier consistency.
5. Enjoy cold straight from the fridge or heat in the microwave for 1-2 minutes if preferred warm.

Nutritional Value (per serving):

> Calories: 280

> Protein: 7g

> Carbohydrates: 42g

> Fat: 10g

> Fiber: 7g

Servings: 1

Difficulty: Easy

Preparation Time: 5 minutes (plus chilling time)

9: Quinoa Breakfast Bowl

Ingredients:

> 1/2 cup cooked quinoa

> 1/4 cup diced mango

> 1/4 cup diced pineapple

> 1 tablespoon unsweetened shredded coconut

> 1 tablespoon chopped almonds

> 1 teaspoon honey or maple syrup (optional)

> 1/4 teaspoon ground cinnamon

Instructions:

1. In a bowl, layer cooked quinoa with diced mango and pineapple.

2. Sprinkle with unsweetened shredded coconut and chopped almonds.

3. Drizzle with honey or maple syrup if desired.

4. Dust with ground cinnamon for added flavor.

5. Mix well before enjoying.

Nutritional Value (per serving):

- Calories: 250
- Protein: 6g
- Carbohydrates: 42g
- Fat: 6g
- Fiber: 6g

Servings: 1

Difficulty: Easy

Preparation Time: 10 minutes

10: Mediterranean Egg Muffins

Ingredients:

- 4 large eggs
- 1/4 cup chopped cherry tomatoes
- 1/4 cup chopped baby spinach
- 2 tablespoons crumbled feta cheese
- 2 tablespoons diced red onion

- ➢ 1/4 teaspoon dried oregano

- ➢ Salt and pepper to taste

- ➢ Cooking spray or olive oil for greasing

Instructions:

1. Preheat the oven to 350°F (175°C). Grease a muffin tin with cooking spray or olive oil.
2. In a bowl, whisk together the eggs until well beaten. Season with salt, pepper, and dried oregano.
3. Divide chopped cherry tomatoes, baby spinach, crumbled feta cheese, and diced red onion evenly among the muffin cups.
4. Pour the beaten eggs over the vegetable mixture in each muffin cup, filling them about 3/4 full.
5. Bake in the preheated oven for 20-25 minutes or until the egg muffins are set and lightly golden on top.
6. Allow the egg muffins to cool slightly before removing them from the muffin tin.
7. Serve warm or at room temperature.

Nutritional Value (per serving - 2 egg muffins):

- ➢ Calories: 180

- ➢ Protein: 14g

- ➢ Carbohydrates: 5g

- ➢ Fat: 12g

- ➢ Fiber: 1g

Servings: 1 (2 egg muffins)

Difficulty: Easy…. Preparation Time: 30 minutes

CHAPTER FIVE: Fatty Liver Lunch Recipes

1: Quinoa and Chickpea Salad

Ingredients:

- 1 cup quinoa
- 1 can (15 oz) chickpeas, drained and rinsed
- 1 cucumber, diced
- 1 bell pepper, diced
- 1/4 cup chopped fresh parsley
- 1/4 cup crumbled feta cheese (optional)
- Juice of 1 lemon
- 2 tablespoons olive oil
- Salt and pepper to taste

Instructions:

1. Cook quinoa according to package instructions. Once cooked, let it cool to room temperature.
2. In a large bowl, combine cooked quinoa, chickpeas, diced cucumber, diced bell pepper, and chopped parsley.
3. In a small bowl, whisk together lemon juice, olive oil, salt, and pepper to make the dressing.
4. Pour the dressing over the quinoa mixture and toss gently to coat.
5. If desired, sprinkle crumbled feta cheese on top before serving.

6.   Divide the salad into two servings and enjoy!

Nutritional Value (per serving):

- ➢ Calories: 380 kcal
- ➢ Protein: 14g
- ➢ Fat: 12g
- ➢ Carbohydrates: 56g
- ➢ Fiber: 11g

Difficulty: Easy

Preparation Time: 20 minutes

2: Grilled Chicken and Vegetable Wrap

Ingredients:

- ➢ 2 boneless, skinless chicken breasts
- ➢ 2 whole wheat tortillas
- ➢ 1 cup mixed salad greens
- ➢ 1 tomato, sliced
- ➢ 1/2 avocado, sliced
- ➢ 1/4 cup shredded carrots
- ➢ 1/4 cup hummus
- ➢ 1 tablespoon olive oil
- ➢ Salt and pepper to taste

Instructions:

1. Preheat grill or grill pan over medium-high heat. Season chicken breasts with olive oil, salt, and pepper.
2. Grill chicken breasts for 6-8 minutes per side or until cooked through. Let them rest for a few minutes before slicing.
3. Warm whole wheat tortillas on the grill for about 30 seconds on each side.
4. Spread hummus evenly over the tortillas.
5. Layer sliced grilled chicken, mixed salad greens, tomato slices, avocado slices, and shredded carrots on top of the hummus.
6. Roll up the tortillas tightly, cut in half, and serve.
7. Repeat for the second wrap.

Nutritional Value (per serving):

- Calories: 420 kcal
- Protein: 32g
- Fat: 18g
- Carbohydrates: 35g
- Fiber: 8g

Difficulty: Moderate

Preparation Time: 30 minutes

3: Salmon and Quinoa Bowl

Ingredients:

- 2 salmon fillets
- 1 cup cooked quinoa
- 1 cup steamed broccoli florets
- 1/2 cup cherry tomatoes, halved
- 1/4 cup diced red onion
- 2 tablespoons chopped fresh dill
- Juice of 1 lemon
- 2 tablespoons olive oil
- Salt and pepper to taste

Instructions:

- Season salmon fillets with salt, pepper, and a drizzle of olive oil. Grill or bake until cooked through, about 10-12 minutes.
- In a bowl, combine cooked quinoa, steamed broccoli, cherry tomatoes, diced red onion, and chopped fresh dill.
- In a small bowl, whisk together lemon juice, olive oil, salt, and pepper to make the dressing.
- Pour the dressing over the quinoa mixture and toss gently to coat.
- Divide the quinoa mixture into two bowls and top each with a grilled salmon fillet.
- Serve immediately.

Nutritional Value (per serving):

- ➢ Calories: 420 kcal
- ➢ Protein: 30g
- ➢ Fat: 20g
- ➢ Carbohydrates: 30g
- ➢ Fiber: 6g

Difficulty: Moderate

Preparation Time: 25 minutes

4: Turkey and Veggie Lettuce Wraps

Ingredients:

- ➢ 8 large lettuce leaves (such as romaine or butter lettuce)
- ➢ 1/2 lb lean ground turkey
- ➢ 1/2 cup diced bell peppers (any color)
- ➢ 1/2 cup shredded carrots
- ➢ 1/4 cup chopped green onions
- ➢ 2 cloves garlic, minced
- ➢ 1 tablespoon soy sauce
- ➢ 1 tablespoon hoisin sauce
- ➢ 1 teaspoon sesame oil
- ➢ 1/4 cup chopped fresh cilantro (optional)

Instructions:

1. Heat a non-stick skillet over medium heat. Add ground turkey and cook until browned, breaking it up with a spoon.
2. Add diced bell peppers, shredded carrots, green onions, and minced garlic to the skillet. Cook for 5-7 minutes, until vegetables are tender.
3. Stir in soy sauce, hoisin sauce, and sesame oil. Cook for an additional 2-3 minutes, stirring occasionally.
4. Spoon the turkey and vegetable mixture onto lettuce leaves. Sprinkle with chopped cilantro, if desired.
5. Roll up the lettuce leaves and serve immediately.

Nutritional Value (per serving, 2 lettuce wraps):

- Calories: 250 kcal
- Protein: 20g
- Fat: 12g
- Carbohydrates: 15g
- Fiber: 5g

Difficulty: Easy

Preparation Time: 20 minutes

5: Veggie Stir-Fry with Tofu

Ingredients:

- ➢ 1 block (14 oz) extra-firm tofu, pressed and cubed
- ➢ 2 cups mixed vegetables (such as bell peppers, broccoli, snap peas, and carrots), sliced
- ➢ 2 tablespoons low-sodium soy sauce
- ➢ 1 tablespoon rice vinegar
- ➢ 1 tablespoon honey or maple syrup
- ➢ 1 teaspoon grated ginger
- ➢ 2 cloves garlic, minced
- ➢ 1 tablespoon sesame oil
- ➢ Cooked brown rice or quinoa, for serving

Instructions:

1. Heat sesame oil in a large skillet or wok over medium-high heat. Add cubed tofu and cook until golden brown on all sides, about 5-7 minutes. Remove tofu from the skillet and set aside.

2. In the same skillet, add a bit more oil if needed, then add mixed vegetables. Stir-fry for 5-7 minutes or until vegetables are tender-crisp.

3. In a small bowl, whisk together soy sauce, rice vinegar, honey or maple syrup, grated ginger, and minced garlic.

4. Return cooked tofu to the skillet, then pour the sauce over the tofu and vegetables. Stir well to coat everything evenly.

5. Cook for another 2-3 minutes until the sauce thickens slightly.

6. Serve the stir-fry over cooked brown rice or quinoa.

Nutritional Value (per serving, without rice/quinoa):

- ➢ Calories: 250 kcal
- ➢ Protein: 18g
- ➢ Fat: 12g
- ➢ Carbohydrates: 20g
- ➢ Fiber: 5g

Difficulty: Moderate

Preparation Time: 30 minutes

6: Mediterranean Chickpea Salad

Ingredients:

- ➢ 1 can (15 oz) chickpeas, drained and rinsed
- ➢ 1 cup diced cucumber
- ➢ 1 cup halved cherry tomatoes
- ➢ 1/4 cup chopped red onion
- ➢ 1/4 cup chopped fresh parsley
- ➢ 2 tablespoons crumbled feta cheese (optional)
- ➢ Juice of 1 lemon
- ➢ 2 tablespoons extra virgin olive oil
- ➢ Salt and pepper to taste

Instructions:

1. In a large bowl, combine chickpeas, diced cucumber, cherry tomatoes, chopped red onion, and chopped parsley.
2. In a small bowl, whisk together lemon juice, olive oil, salt, and pepper to make the dressing.
3. Pour the dressing over the chickpea mixture and toss gently to coat.
4. If desired, sprinkle crumbled feta cheese on top before serving.
5. Divide the salad into two servings and enjoy!

Nutritional Value (per serving):

➢ Calories: 280 kcal
➢ Protein: 10g
➢ Fat: 14g
➢ Carbohydrates: 30g
➢ Fiber: 9g

Difficulty: Easy

Preparation Time: 15 minutes

7: Lentil and Vegetable Soup

Ingredients:

➢ 1 cup dried green lentils, rinsed
➢ 4 cups vegetable broth

- 1 onion, diced
- 2 carrots, diced
- 2 celery stalks, diced
- 2 cloves garlic, minced
- 1 teaspoon ground cumin
- 1 teaspoon paprika
- Salt and pepper to taste
- Fresh parsley for garnish (optional)

Instructions:

1. In a large pot, sauté diced onion, carrots, and celery over medium heat until softened, about 5 minutes.
2. Add minced garlic, ground cumin, and paprika to the pot. Cook for another minute until fragrant.
3. Add rinsed lentils and vegetable broth to the pot. Bring to a boil, then reduce heat and simmer for 20-25 minutes, or until lentils are tender.
4. Season with salt and pepper to taste.
5. Ladle the soup into bowls and garnish with fresh parsley if desired.
6. Serve hot and enjoy!

Nutritional Value (per serving):

- Calories: 220 kcal
- Protein: 13g

- ➤ Fat: 1g

- ➤ Carbohydrates: 40g

- ➤ Fiber: 15g

Difficulty: Easy

Preparation Time: 30 minutes

8: Turkey and Quinoa Stuffed Bell Peppers

Ingredients:

- ➤ 4 bell peppers, halved and seeds removed

- ➤ 1 cup cooked quinoa

- ➤ 1/2 lb lean ground turkey

- ➤ 1 onion, diced

- ➤ 1 zucchini, diced

- ➤ 1 tomato, diced

- ➤ 2 cloves garlic, minced

- ➤ 1 teaspoon dried oregano

- ➤ 1 teaspoon dried basil

- ➤ Salt and pepper to taste

- ➤ 1/2 cup shredded mozzarella cheese (optional)

Instructions:

- ➤ Preheat oven to 375°F (190°C). Place halved bell peppers in a baking dish.

- In a skillet, cook ground turkey over medium heat until browned. Add diced onion, zucchini, tomato, and minced garlic. Cook until vegetables are tender.
- Stir in cooked quinoa, dried oregano, dried basil, salt, and pepper. Cook for another 2-3 minutes.
- Spoon the turkey and quinoa mixture into each bell pepper half.
- If desired, sprinkle shredded mozzarella cheese on top of each stuffed pepper.
- Cover the baking dish with foil and bake for 25-30 minutes, or until peppers are tender.
- Serve hot and enjoy!

Nutritional Value (per serving, 2 stuffed pepper halves):

- Calories: 320 kcal
- Protein: 25g
- Fat: 8g
- Carbohydrates: 35g
- Fiber: 8g

Difficulty: Moderate

Preparation Time: 45 minutes

9: Avocado and Black Bean Quesadillas

Ingredients:

- ➤ 4 whole grain or corn tortillas
- ➤ 1 ripe avocado, mashed
- ➤ 1 cup cooked black beans, drained and rinsed
- ➤ 1/2 cup diced tomatoes
- ➤ 1/4 cup chopped fresh cilantro
- ➤ 1/2 cup shredded reduced-fat cheddar cheese
- ➤ 1 tablespoon lime juice
- ➤ 1 teaspoon ground cumin
- ➤ 1/2 teaspoon chili powder
- ➤ Salt and pepper to taste
- ➤ Cooking spray

Instructions:

1. In a bowl, mix together mashed avocado, black beans, diced tomatoes, chopped cilantro, lime juice, ground cumin, chili powder, salt, and pepper.
2. Lay out half of the tortillas and spread the avocado and black bean mixture evenly over each one.
3. Sprinkle shredded cheese over the mixture and place the remaining tortillas on top to create quesadillas.
4. Heat a large skillet over medium heat and lightly coat with cooking spray.

5. Carefully transfer each quesadilla to the skillet and cook for 2-3 minutes on each side, or until golden brown and crispy.

6. Once cooked, remove from the skillet and cut into wedges.

7. Serve hot with salsa, Greek yogurt, or your favorite dipping sauce.

Nutritional Value (per serving, 1 quesadilla):

- Calories: 280 kcal
- Protein: 12g
- Fat: 12g
- Carbohydrates: 30g
- Fiber: 8g

Difficulty: Moderate

Preparation Time: 20 minutes

10: Mediterranean Chickpea Wraps

Ingredients:

- 4 whole grain wraps or large lettuce leaves
- 1 can (15 oz) chickpeas, drained and rinsed
- 1/2 cup diced cucumber
- 1/2 cup halved cherry tomatoes
- 1/4 cup diced red onion
- 1/4 cup chopped fresh parsley
- Juice of 1 lemon

- ➢ 2 tablespoons extra virgin olive oil

- ➢ Salt and pepper to taste

- ➢ Hummus or tzatziki sauce for spreading

Instructions:

1. In a bowl, combine chickpeas, diced cucumber, cherry tomatoes, diced red onion, chopped parsley, lemon juice, olive oil, salt, and pepper. Mix well to combine.
2. Warm the wraps or lettuce leaves slightly to make them more pliable.
3. Spread a layer of hummus or tzatziki sauce onto each wrap or lettuce leaf.
4. Spoon the chickpea mixture onto the wraps or lettuce leaves, distributing evenly.
5. Roll up the wraps or lettuce leaves tightly, tucking in the sides as you go.
6. If using wraps, slice each wrap in half diagonally. If using lettuce leaves, simply serve as wraps.
7. Serve immediately, or wrap in foil or parchment paper for a portable lunch option.

Nutritional Value (per serving, 1 wrap):

- ➢ Calories: 280 kcal

- ➢ Protein: 10g

- ➢ Fat: 10g

> Carbohydrates: 40g

> Fiber: 10g

Difficulty: Easy

Preparation Time: 15 minutes

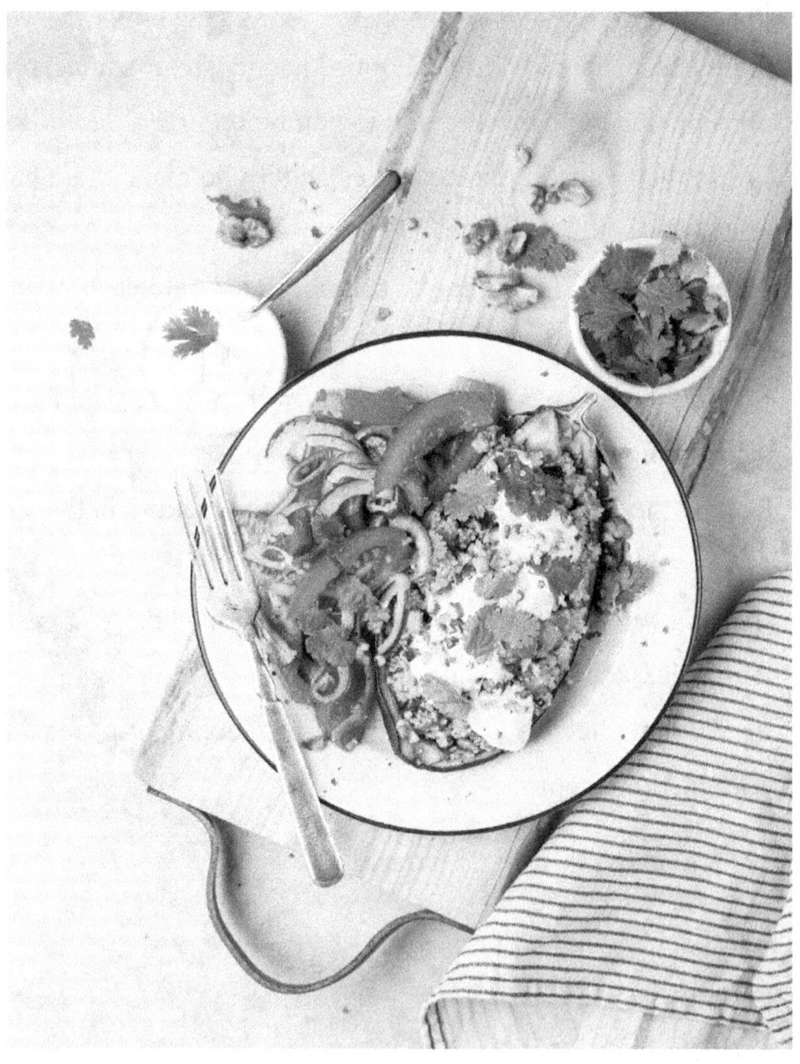

CHAPTER SIX: Fatty Liver Dinner Recipes

1. Grilled Lemon Herb Chicken with Roasted Vegetables

Ingredients:

- 4 boneless, skinless chicken breasts
- 2 tablespoons olive oil
- 2 cloves garlic, minced
- 1 tablespoon lemon zest
- 2 tablespoons fresh lemon juice
- 1 teaspoon dried thyme
- 1 teaspoon dried rosemary
- Salt and pepper to taste
- 2 cups mixed vegetables (such as bell peppers, zucchini, and cherry tomatoes)
- Cooking spray

Instructions:

1. In a small bowl, whisk together olive oil, minced garlic, lemon zest, lemon juice, thyme, rosemary, salt, and pepper.
2. Place chicken breasts in a shallow dish and pour the marinade over them. Let marinate in the refrigerator for at least 30 minutes.

3. Preheat grill to medium-high heat. Remove chicken from marinade and discard excess marinade.

4. Grill chicken for 6-8 minutes per side or until cooked through and no longer pink in the center.

5. Meanwhile, toss mixed vegetables with a little olive oil, salt, and pepper. Spread them out on a baking sheet lined with parchment paper.

6. Roast vegetables in the oven at 400°F (200°C) for 15-20 minutes or until tender and slightly charred.

7. Serve grilled chicken with roasted vegetables.

Nutritional Value (per serving):

➢ Calories: 300 kcal

➢ Protein: 30g

➢ Carbohydrates: 10g

➢ Fat: 15g

➢ Fiber: 4g

Difficulty: Easy

Servings: 4

Preparation Time: 40 minutes

2: Baked Salmon with Lemon Dill Sauce

Ingredients:

- ➢ 4 salmon fillets
- ➢ 2 tablespoons olive oil
- ➢ Salt and pepper to taste
- ➢ 2 tablespoons chopped fresh dill
- ➢ 1 tablespoon lemon juice
- ➢ 1 teaspoon Dijon mustard
- ➢ 2 tablespoons Greek yogurt
- ➢ 1 garlic clove, minced
- ➢ Lemon slices for garnish

Instructions:

- ➢ Preheat oven to 375°F (190°C). Place salmon fillets on a baking sheet lined with parchment paper. Drizzle with olive oil and season with salt and pepper.
- ➢ Bake salmon for 12-15 minutes or until fish flakes easily with a fork.
- ➢ While salmon is baking, prepare the lemon dill sauce. In a small bowl, whisk together chopped dill, lemon juice, Dijon mustard, Greek yogurt, minced garlic, salt, and pepper.
- ➢ Serve baked salmon with lemon dill sauce drizzled on top. Garnish with lemon slices.

Nutritional Value (per serving):

> Calories: 300 kcal

> Protein: 25g

> Carbohydrates: 2g

> Fat: 20g

> Fiber: 0g

Difficulty: Easy

Servings: 4

Preparation Time: 20 minutes

3: Turkey and Vegetable Stir-Fry

Ingredients:

> 1 lb lean ground turkey

> 2 tablespoons low-sodium soy sauce

> 1 tablespoon rice vinegar

> 1 teaspoon sesame oil

> 2 cloves garlic, minced

> 1 tablespoon grated ginger

> 2 cups mixed vegetables (such as bell peppers, broccoli, and snap peas)

> 2 green onions, chopped

> 2 cups cooked brown rice

> Cooking spray

Instructions:

1. Heat a large skillet or wok over medium-high heat. Spray with cooking spray and add ground turkey. Cook until browned and cooked through.
2. In a small bowl, mix together soy sauce, rice vinegar, and sesame oil.
3. Push turkey to one side of the skillet and add minced garlic and grated ginger. Cook for 1 minute until fragrant.
4. Add mixed vegetables to the skillet and stir-fry until tender-crisp.
5. Pour the soy sauce mixture over the turkey and vegetables. Stir to combine and cook for another 2-3 minutes.
6. Serve turkey and vegetable stir-fry over cooked brown rice. Garnish with chopped green onions.

Nutritional Value (per serving):

- Calories: 350 kcal
- Protein: 25g
- Carbohydrates: 40g
- Fat: 10g
- Fiber: 6g

Difficulty: Moderate

Servings: 4

Preparation Time: 30 minutes

4: Lentil and Vegetable Curry

Ingredients:

- ➢ 1 cup dried green lentils
- ➢ 2 cups vegetable broth
- ➢ 1 tablespoon olive oil
- ➢ 1 onion, diced
- ➢ 2 cloves garlic, minced
- ➢ 1 tablespoon grated ginger
- ➢ 2 tablespoons curry powder
- ➢ 1 teaspoon ground cumin
- ➢ 1 teaspoon ground coriander
- ➢ 1 can (14 oz) diced tomatoes
- ➢ 2 cups mixed vegetables (such as cauliflower, carrots, and spinach)
- ➢ Salt and pepper to taste
- ➢ Fresh cilantro for garnish
- ➢ Cooked quinoa or brown rice for serving

Instructions:

1. Rinse lentils under cold water and drain. In a medium saucepan, combine lentils and vegetable broth. Bring to a boil,

then reduce heat to low and simmer for 20-25 minutes or until lentils are tender.

2. In a large skillet, heat olive oil over medium heat. Add diced onion and cook until softened. Add minced garlic and grated ginger, and cook for another minute until fragrant.

3. Stir in curry powder, ground cumin, and ground coriander, and cook for 1-2 minutes until spices are toasted.

4. Add diced tomatoes (with juices) to the skillet and stir to combine. Cook for 5 minutes, allowing the flavors to meld.

5. Add mixed vegetables to the skillet and cooked lentils with their cooking liquid. Simmer for 10-15 minutes or until vegetables are tender.

6. Season with salt and pepper to taste. Serve lentil and vegetable curry over cooked quinoa or brown rice. Garnish with fresh cilantro.

Nutritional Value (per serving):

➤ Calories: 320 kcal

➤ Protein: 18g

➤ Carbohydrates: 50g

➤ Fat: 6g

➤ Fiber: 12g

Difficulty: Moderate

Servings: 4

Preparation Time: 45 minutes

5: Quinoa Stuffed Bell Peppers

Ingredients:

- 4 bell peppers (any color)
- 1 cup quinoa, rinsed
- 2 cups vegetable broth
- 1 tablespoon olive oil
- 1 onion, diced
- 2 cloves garlic, minced
- 1 zucchini, diced
- 1 tomato, diced
- 1 cup canned black beans, drained and rinsed
- 1 teaspoon ground cumin
- 1 teaspoon paprika
- Salt and pepper to taste
- Fresh cilantro for garnish

Instructions:

1. Preheat oven to 375°F (190°C). Slice the tops off the bell peppers and remove the seeds and membranes. Place the peppers in a baking dish.

2. In a saucepan, bring vegetable broth to a boil. Add quinoa, reduce heat to low, cover, and simmer for 15-20 minutes or until quinoa is cooked and liquid is absorbed.

3. In a large skillet, heat olive oil over medium heat. Add diced onion and cook until softened. Add minced garlic and cook for another minute until fragrant.

4. Add diced zucchini and tomato to the skillet and cook until vegetables are tender.

5. Stir in cooked quinoa, black beans, ground cumin, paprika, salt, and pepper. Cook for 5 minutes, allowing flavors to meld.

6. Spoon quinoa mixture into each bell pepper until filled. Cover the baking dish with foil and bake for 25-30 minutes or until peppers are tender.

7. Serve quinoa stuffed bell peppers garnished with fresh cilantro.

Nutritional Value (per serving):

➢ Calories: 320 kcal

➢ Protein: 12g

➢ Carbohydrates: 55g

➢ Fat: 7g

➢ Fiber: 12g

Difficulty: Moderate

Servings: 4

Preparation Time: 50 minutes

6: Garlic Shrimp with Lemon Zucchini Noodles

Ingredients:

- 1 lb large shrimp, peeled and deveined
- 3 tablespoons olive oil
- 4 cloves garlic, minced
- Zest and juice of 1 lemon
- 4 medium zucchini, spiralized into noodles
- Salt and pepper to taste
- Red pepper flakes (optional)
- Fresh parsley for garnish

Instructions:

1. In a large skillet, heat 2 tablespoons of olive oil over medium heat. Add minced garlic and cook for 1 minute until fragrant.
2. Add shrimp to the skillet and cook for 2-3 minutes on each side until pink and cooked through. Remove shrimp from the skillet and set aside.
3. In the same skillet, add remaining olive oil and lemon zest. Add spiralized zucchini noodles and cook for 2-3 minutes until tender but still crisp.

4. Return cooked shrimp to the skillet. Add lemon juice, salt, pepper, and red pepper flakes if using. Toss everything together until heated through.

5. Serve garlic shrimp with lemon zucchini noodles garnished with fresh parsley.

Nutritional Value (per serving):

- Calories: 250 kcal
- Protein: 25g
- Carbohydrates: 10g
- Fat: 14g
- Fiber: 3g

Difficulty: Easy

Servings: 4

Preparation Time: 25 minutes

7: Baked Cod with Mediterranean Salsa

Ingredients:

- 4 cod fillets
- 2 tablespoons olive oil
- 2 cloves garlic, minced
- 1 teaspoon dried oregano
- 1 teaspoon dried basil

- ➢ Salt and pepper to taste
- ➢ 1 cup cherry tomatoes, halved
- ➢ 1/2 cucumber, diced
- ➢ 1/4 red onion, finely chopped
- ➢ 1/4 cup Kalamata olives, chopped
- ➢ 2 tablespoons fresh lemon juice
- ➢ 2 tablespoons chopped fresh parsley

Instructions:

1. Preheat oven to 375°F (190°C). Place cod fillets on a baking sheet lined with parchment paper.
2. In a small bowl, mix together olive oil, minced garlic, dried oregano, dried basil, salt, and pepper.
3. Brush the olive oil mixture over the cod fillets.
4. Bake cod in the preheated oven for 15-20 minutes or until fish flakes easily with a fork.
5. In the meantime, prepare the Mediterranean salsa. In a bowl, combine cherry tomatoes, diced cucumber, red onion, chopped olives, lemon juice, and chopped parsley.
6. Serve baked cod with Mediterranean salsa on top.

Nutritional Value (per serving):

- ➢ Calories: 250 kcal
- ➢ Protein: 30g
- ➢ Carbohydrates: 7g

- ➢ Fat: 11g
- ➢ Fiber: 2g

Difficulty: Easy

Servings: 4

Preparation Time: 25 minutes

8: Tofu and Vegetable Coconut Curry

Ingredients:

- ➢ 1 tablespoon coconut oil
- ➢ 1 onion, diced
- ➢ 2 cloves garlic, minced
- ➢ 1 tablespoon grated ginger
- ➢ 1 tablespoon red curry paste
- ➢ 1 can (14 oz) coconut milk
- ➢ 2 cups mixed vegetables (such as bell peppers, broccoli, and carrots)
- ➢ 1 block (14 oz) firm tofu, cubed
- ➢ 1 tablespoon soy sauce
- ➢ 1 tablespoon lime juice
- ➢ Salt and pepper to taste
- ➢ Cooked brown rice for serving

Instructions:

1. Heat coconut oil in a large skillet over medium heat. Add diced onion and cook until softened.
2. Add minced garlic and grated ginger to the skillet. Cook for another minute until fragrant.
3. Stir in red curry paste and cook for 1-2 minutes.
4. Pour coconut milk into the skillet and bring to a simmer.
5. Add mixed vegetables and cubed tofu to the skillet. Cook until vegetables are tender and tofu is heated through.
6. Stir in soy sauce and lime juice. Season with salt and pepper to taste.
7. Serve tofu and vegetable coconut curry over cooked brown rice.

Nutritional Value (per serving):

- Calories: 300 kcal
- Protein: 15g
- Carbohydrates: 20g
- Fat: 20g
- Fiber: 5g

Difficulty: Moderate

Servings: 4

Preparation Time: 30 minutes

9: Baked Turkey Meatballs with Zucchini Noodles

Ingredients:

- 1 lb lean ground turkey
- 1/4 cup breadcrumbs (use whole wheat for added fiber)
- 1 egg, lightly beaten
- 2 cloves garlic, minced
- 1/4 cup grated Parmesan cheese
- 1 teaspoon dried oregano
- 1 teaspoon dried basil
- Salt and pepper to taste
- 4 medium zucchini, spiralized into noodles
- 2 cups marinara sauce (use low-sodium and sugar-free if possible)
- Cooking spray

Instructions:

1. Preheat oven to 375°F (190°C). Line a baking sheet with parchment paper and lightly coat it with cooking spray.
2. In a large bowl, combine ground turkey, breadcrumbs, beaten egg, minced garlic, grated Parmesan cheese, dried oregano, dried basil, salt, and pepper. Mix until well combined.
3. Roll the turkey mixture into meatballs (about 1 inch in diameter) and place them on the prepared baking sheet.

4. Bake meatballs in the preheated oven for 20-25 minutes or until cooked through and lightly browned.

5. In a separate skillet, heat marinara sauce over medium heat until heated through.

6. While the meatballs are baking, heat a little olive oil in another skillet over medium heat. Add spiralized zucchini noodles and cook for 2-3 minutes until tender but still crisp.

7. Serve baked turkey meatballs over zucchini noodles, topped with marinara sauce.

Nutritional Value (per serving):

➢ Calories: 300 kcal

➢ Protein: 25g

➢ Carbohydrates: 15g

➢ Fat: 15g

➢ Fiber: 4g

Difficulty: Easy

Servings: 4

Preparation Time: 40 minutes

10: Salmon and Asparagus Foil Packets

Ingredients:

➢ 4 salmon fillets

- 1 bunch asparagus, trimmed
- 2 tablespoons olive oil
- 2 cloves garlic, minced
- 1 lemon, thinly sliced
- Salt and pepper to taste
- Fresh dill for garnish

Instructions:

1. Preheat oven to 400°F (200°C). Cut four large pieces of aluminum foil.
2. Place a salmon fillet on each piece of foil. Arrange trimmed asparagus around the salmon.
3. Drizzle olive oil over the salmon and asparagus. Sprinkle minced garlic on top. Season with salt and pepper to taste.
4. Place lemon slices on top of each salmon fillet.
5. Fold the sides of the foil over the salmon and asparagus, sealing to form a packet.
6. Place foil packets on a baking sheet and bake in the preheated oven for 15-20 minutes or until salmon is cooked through and asparagus is tender.
7. Carefully open the foil packets and transfer salmon and asparagus to plates. Garnish with fresh dill before serving.

Nutritional Value (per serving):

- Calories: 300 kcal

> Protein: 25g

> Carbohydrates: 8g

> Fat: 18g

> Fiber: 3g

Difficulty: Easy

Servings: 4

Preparation Time: 25 minutes

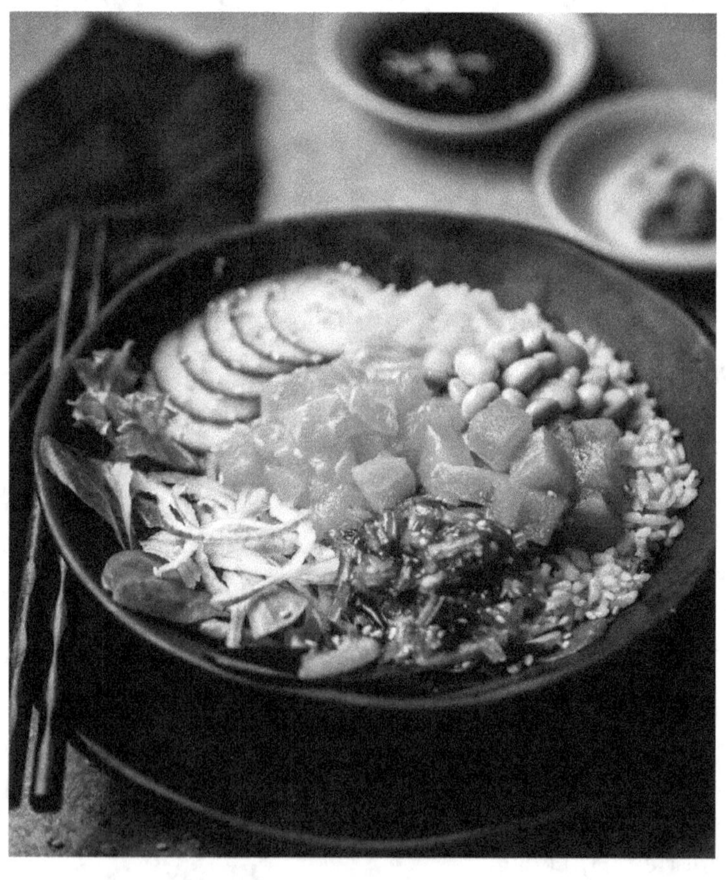

CHAPTER SEVEN: Fatty Liver Grain & Legumes Recipes

1: Quinoa and Black Bean Stuffed Bell Peppers

Ingredients:

- 4 large bell peppers (any color)
- 1 cup quinoa, rinsed
- 1 can (15 ounces) black beans, drained and rinsed
- 1 cup diced tomatoes
- 1/2 cup diced red onion
- 2 cloves garlic, minced
- 1 teaspoon ground cumin
- 1 teaspoon chili powder
- Salt and pepper, to taste
- 1 cup shredded cheddar cheese (optional)
- Fresh cilantro, for garnish

Instructions:

1. Preheat the oven to 375°F (190°C). Cut the tops off the bell peppers and remove the seeds and membranes.
2. In a large bowl, mix together quinoa, black beans, diced tomatoes, red onion, garlic, cumin, chili powder, salt, and pepper.
3. Stuff each bell pepper with the quinoa and black bean mixture.

4. Place the stuffed bell peppers in a baking dish. If using cheese, sprinkle it on top of the stuffed peppers.

5. Cover the baking dish with aluminum foil and bake for 30-35 minutes, or until the peppers are tender.

6. Remove the foil and bake for an additional 5-10 minutes, or until the cheese is melted and bubbly.

7. Garnish with fresh cilantro before serving.

Nutritional Value (per serving):

➢ Calories: 320 kcal

➢ Protein: 14g

➢ Carbohydrates: 49g

➢ Fat: 7g

➢ Fiber: 10g

Servings: 4

Difficulty: Medium

Preparation Time: 40 minutes

2: Lentil and Vegetable Stir-Fry with Brown Rice

Ingredients:

➢ 1 cup brown lentils, rinsed

➢ 2 cups vegetable broth

➢ 2 tablespoons soy sauce (or tamari for gluten-free)

- ➢ 1 tablespoon sesame oil
- ➢ 2 cloves garlic, minced
- ➢ 1 teaspoon grated ginger
- ➢ 2 cups mixed vegetables (such as bell peppers, broccoli, carrots, snap peas)
- ➢ Cooked brown rice, for serving
- ➢ Sesame seeds, for garnish (optional)
- ➢ Green onions, sliced, for garnish (optional)

Instructions:

1. In a medium saucepan, combine lentils and vegetable broth. Bring to a boil, then reduce heat, cover, and simmer for 20-25 minutes, or until lentils are tender.
2. In a small bowl, mix together soy sauce and sesame oil. Set aside.
3. Heat a large skillet or wok over medium-high heat. Add garlic and ginger, and cook for 1-2 minutes until fragrant.
4. Add mixed vegetables to the skillet and stir-fry for 5-7 minutes, or until vegetables are tender-crisp.
5. Add cooked lentils to the skillet, along with the soy sauce mixture. Stir-fry for an additional 2-3 minutes to combine flavors.
6. Serve the lentil and vegetable stir-fry over cooked brown rice.
7. Garnish with sesame seeds and sliced green onions, if desired.

Nutritional Value (per serving):

> Calories: 320 kcal

> Protein: 15g

> Carbohydrates: 55g

> Fat: 4g

> Fiber: 12g

Servings: 4

Difficulty: Easy

Preparation Time: 30 minutes

3: Chickpea and Vegetable Curry with Quinoa

Ingredients:

> 1 cup quinoa, rinsed

> 1 tablespoon coconut oil

> 1 onion, diced

> 2 cloves garlic, minced

> 1 tablespoon grated ginger

> 2 teaspoons curry powder

> 1 teaspoon ground turmeric

> 1 can (15 ounces) chickpeas, drained and rinsed

> 1 can (14 ounces) diced tomatoes

> 1 can (14 ounces) coconut milk

- ➢ 2 cups mixed vegetables (such as cauliflower, bell peppers, and spinach)
- ➢ Salt and pepper, to taste
- ➢ Fresh cilantro, for garnish
- ➢ Cooked quinoa, for serving

Instructions:

1. In a saucepan, cook quinoa according to package instructions. Set aside.
2. In a large skillet, heat coconut oil over medium heat. Add diced onion and cook until softened, about 5 minutes.
3. Add minced garlic, grated ginger, curry powder, and turmeric to the skillet. Cook for 1-2 minutes until fragrant.
4. Stir in chickpeas, diced tomatoes, and coconut milk. Bring to a simmer and let it cook for 10-15 minutes, allowing flavors to meld.
5. Add mixed vegetables to the skillet and cook until tender, about 5-7 minutes.
6. Season with salt and pepper to taste.
7. Serve the chickpea and vegetable curry over cooked quinoa.
8. Garnish with fresh cilantro before serving.

Nutritional Value (per serving):

- ➢ Calories: 380 kcal
- ➢ Protein: 12g

- ➢ Carbohydrates: 48g

- ➢ Fat: 18g

- ➢ Fiber: 10g

- ➢ Servings: 4

Difficulty: Medium

Preparation Time: 30 minutes

4: Lentil and Sweet Potato Shepherd's Pie

Ingredients:

- ➢ 2 large sweet potatoes, peeled and cubed

- ➢ 1 tablespoon olive oil

- ➢ 1 onion, diced

- ➢ 2 cloves garlic, minced

- ➢ 2 carrots, diced

- ➢ 2 celery stalks, diced

- ➢ 1 cup green lentils, rinsed

- ➢ 2 cups vegetable broth

- ➢ 1 teaspoon dried thyme

- ➢ Salt and pepper, to taste

- ➢ Fresh parsley, for garnish

- ➢ Cooked quinoa, for serving

Instructions:

1. Preheat the oven to 375°F (190°C). Place sweet potato cubes in a pot of boiling water and cook until tender, about 10-15 minutes. Drain and set aside.
2. In a large skillet, heat olive oil over medium heat. Add diced onion and cook until softened, about 5 minutes.
3. Add minced garlic, diced carrots, and diced celery to the skillet. Cook for another 5 minutes until vegetables are tender.
4. Stir in green lentils, vegetable broth, dried thyme, salt, and pepper. Bring to a boil, then reduce heat and simmer for 20-25 minutes, or until lentils are cooked through and most of the liquid is absorbed.
5. Mash the cooked sweet potatoes with a fork until smooth.
6. Transfer the lentil mixture to a baking dish. Spread mashed sweet potatoes on top.
7. Bake in the preheated oven for 20-25 minutes, or until the top is golden brown.
8. Garnish with fresh parsley before serving.
9. Serve the lentil and sweet potato shepherd's pie over cooked quinoa.

Nutritional Value (per serving):

➤ Calories: 340 kcal
➤ Protein: 12g

- ➤ Carbohydrates: 60g
- ➤ Fat: 5g
- ➤ Fiber: 12g

Servings: 4

Difficulty: Medium

Preparation Time: 50 minutes

5: Brown Rice and Black Bean Burrito Bowls

Ingredients:

- ➤ 1 cup brown rice
- ➤ 1 can (15 ounces) black beans, drained and rinsed
- ➤ 1 cup corn kernels (fresh, frozen, or canned)
- ➤ 1 red bell pepper, diced
- ➤ 1 avocado, diced
- ➤ 1/4 cup chopped fresh cilantro
- ➤ 1 lime, juiced
- ➤ 1 teaspoon ground cumin
- ➤ 1/2 teaspoon chili powder
- ➤ Salt and pepper, to taste
- ➤ Optional toppings: salsa, Greek yogurt or sour cream, shredded cheese

Instructions:

1. Cook brown rice according to package instructions.
2. In a large skillet, heat black beans and corn over medium heat. Add diced red bell pepper, ground cumin, chili powder, salt, and pepper. Cook for 5-7 minutes, stirring occasionally.
3. In a small bowl, combine diced avocado, chopped cilantro, and lime juice.
4. To assemble the burrito bowls, divide cooked brown rice among serving bowls. Top with the black bean and corn mixture, avocado salsa, and any optional toppings of your choice.
5. Serve immediately and enjoy!

Nutritional Value (per serving):

➢ Calories: 380 kcal
➢ Protein: 12g
➢ Carbohydrates: 64g
➢ Fat: 10g
➢ Fiber: 12g

Servings: 4

Difficulty: Easy

Preparation Time: 20 minutes

Ingredients:

- 1 cup quinoa, rinsed
- 1/2 cup green or brown lentils, rinsed
- 2 cups water or vegetable broth
- 1 cucumber, diced
- 1 bell pepper, diced
- 1/4 cup chopped fresh parsley
- 1/4 cup chopped fresh mint
- 1/4 cup crumbled feta cheese (optional)
- 1 lemon, juiced
- 2 tablespoons extra-virgin olive oil
- 1 teaspoon honey or maple syrup (optional)
- Salt and pepper, to taste

Instructions:

1. In a medium saucepan, combine quinoa, lentils, and water or vegetable broth. Bring to a boil, then reduce heat, cover, and simmer for 15-20 minutes, or until quinoa and lentils are cooked and liquid is absorbed. Remove from heat and let it cool slightly.

2. In a large bowl, combine cooked quinoa and lentils with diced cucumber, bell pepper, chopped parsley, chopped mint, and crumbled feta cheese (if using).

3. In a small bowl, whisk together lemon juice, olive oil, honey or maple syrup (if using), salt, and pepper to make the dressing.

4. Pour the dressing over the quinoa and lentil mixture and toss gently to coat.

5. Serve the quinoa and lentil salad at room temperature or chilled.

6. Enjoy as a light and refreshing meal or side dish!

Nutritional Value (per serving):

➢ Calories: 320 kcal

➢ Protein: 12g

➢ Carbohydrates: 45g

➢ Fat: 10g

➢ Fiber: 8g

Servings: 4

Difficulty: Easy

Preparation Time: 20 minutes

7: Barley and Vegetable Soup

Ingredients:

➢ 1 cup pearl barley, rinsed

➢ 6 cups vegetable broth

- ➢ 1 onion, diced
- ➢ 2 carrots, diced
- ➢ 2 celery stalks, diced
- ➢ 2 cloves garlic, minced
- ➢ 1 can (15 ounces) diced tomatoes
- ➢ 1 can (15 ounces) kidney beans, drained and rinsed
- ➢ 1 teaspoon dried thyme
- ➢ 1 teaspoon dried rosemary
- ➢ Salt and pepper, to taste
- ➢ Fresh parsley, for garnish

Instructions:

1. In a large pot, combine pearl barley and vegetable broth. Bring to a boil, then reduce heat and simmer for 30 minutes.
2. In a separate pan, heat olive oil over medium heat. Add diced onion, carrots, celery, and minced garlic. Cook until vegetables are softened, about 5-7 minutes.
3. Add the cooked vegetables to the pot with barley and broth.
4. Stir in diced tomatoes, kidney beans, dried thyme, dried rosemary, salt, and pepper.
5. Continue to simmer the soup for an additional 15-20 minutes, or until barley is tender and flavors are well combined.
6. Adjust seasoning if necessary.
7. Serve hot, garnished with fresh parsley.

Nutritional Value (per serving):

- ➤ Calories: 280 kcal
- ➤ Protein: 10g
- ➤ Carbohydrates: 55g
- ➤ Fat: 1g
- ➤ Fiber: 12g
- ➤ Servings: 6

Difficulty: Easy

Preparation Time: 60 minutes

8: Lentil and Mushroom Stir-Fry with Quinoa

Ingredients:

- ➤ 1 cup quinoa, rinsed
- ➤ 2 cups water or vegetable broth
- ➤ 1 tablespoon olive oil
- ➤ 1 onion, sliced
- ➤ 2 cloves garlic, minced
- ➤ 8 ounces mushrooms, sliced
- ➤ 1 can (15 ounces) lentils, drained and rinsed
- ➤ 2 tablespoons soy sauce or tamari
- ➤ 1 teaspoon sesame oil
- ➤ 1 teaspoon sriracha sauce (optional)
- ➤ 2 cups baby spinach

➢ Salt and pepper, to taste

➢ Sesame seeds, for garnish

Instructions:

1. In a saucepan, combine quinoa and water or vegetable broth. Bring to a boil, then reduce heat, cover, and simmer for 15-20 minutes, or until quinoa is cooked and liquid is absorbed. Set aside.

2. In a large skillet or wok, heat olive oil over medium-high heat. Add sliced onion and cook until softened, about 3-4 minutes.

3. Add minced garlic and sliced mushrooms to the skillet. Cook for another 5-7 minutes, or until mushrooms are golden brown.

4. Stir in drained lentils, soy sauce or tamari, sesame oil, and sriracha sauce (if using). Cook for 2-3 minutes, allowing flavors to meld.

5. Add baby spinach to the skillet and cook until wilted, about 1-2 minutes.

6. Season with salt and pepper to taste.

7. Serve the lentil and mushroom stir-fry over cooked quinoa.

8. Garnish with sesame seeds before serving.

Nutritional Value (per serving):

➢ Calories: 320 kcal

➢ Protein: 14g

➢ Carbohydrates: 45g

- ➢ Fat: 8g
- ➢ Fiber: 10g

Servings: 4

Difficulty: Easy

Preparation Time: 30 minutes

9: Millet and Chickpea Buddha Bowl

Ingredients:

- ➢ 1 cup millet, rinsed
- ➢ 2 cups vegetable broth
- ➢ 1 can (15 ounces) chickpeas, drained and rinsed
- ➢ 2 cups mixed greens (such as spinach, kale, and arugula)
- ➢ 1 cup cherry tomatoes, halved
- ➢ 1 cucumber, diced
- ➢ 1 avocado, sliced
- ➢ 1/4 cup sliced almonds
- ➢ 2 tablespoons lemon juice
- ➢ 2 tablespoons extra-virgin olive oil
- ➢ 1 teaspoon Dijon mustard
- ➢ Salt and pepper, to taste

Instructions:

1. In a saucepan, combine millet and vegetable broth. Bring to a boil, then reduce heat, cover, and simmer for 20-25 minutes, or until millet is cooked and liquid is absorbed. Fluff with a fork and let it cool slightly.
2. In a large bowl, assemble mixed greens, halved cherry tomatoes, diced cucumber, sliced avocado, and cooked chickpeas.
3. In a small bowl, whisk together lemon juice, olive oil, Dijon mustard, salt, and pepper to make the dressing.
4. Add cooked millet to the bowl of mixed greens and vegetables.
5. Drizzle the dressing over the Buddha bowl and toss gently to coat.
6. Sprinkle sliced almonds on top before serving.
7. Enjoy this nutritious and flavorful Buddha bowl!

Nutritional Value (per serving):

- Calories: 380 kcal
- Protein: 12g
- Carbohydrates: 50g
- Fat: 15g
- Fiber: 10g

Servings: 4

Difficulty: Easy

Preparation Time: 25 minutes

10: Wild Rice and Lentil Stuffed Bell Peppers

Ingredients:

- 4 large bell peppers (any color)
- 1 cup wild rice, rinsed
- 1/2 cup green or brown lentils, rinsed
- 2 cups vegetable broth
- 1 onion, diced
- 2 cloves garlic, minced
- 1 carrot, diced
- 1 stalk celery, diced
- 1 can (15 ounces) diced tomatoes
- 1 teaspoon dried oregano
- 1 teaspoon dried basil
- Salt and pepper, to taste
- Fresh parsley, for garnish

Instructions:

1. Preheat the oven to 375°F (190°C). Cut the tops off the bell peppers and remove the seeds and membranes.
2. In a saucepan, combine wild rice, lentils, and vegetable broth. Bring to a boil, then reduce heat, cover, and simmer for 30-35

minutes, or until rice and lentils are tender and liquid is absorbed.

3. In a large skillet, heat olive oil over medium heat. Add diced onion, minced garlic, diced carrot, and diced celery. Cook until vegetables are softened, about 5-7 minutes.

4. Stir in diced tomatoes, dried oregano, dried basil, salt, and pepper. Cook for another 2-3 minutes, allowing flavors to meld.

5. Add cooked wild rice and lentils to the skillet. Stir to combine.

6. Stuff each bell pepper with the wild rice and lentil mixture.

7. Place stuffed bell peppers in a baking dish. Cover with aluminum foil and bake for 25-30 minutes, or until peppers are tender.

8. Garnish with fresh parsley before serving.

9. Serve these hearty and satisfying stuffed bell peppers as a nutritious meal!

Nutritional Value (per serving):

➢ Calories: 320 kcal

➢ Protein: 10g

➢ Carbohydrates: 60g

➢ Fat: 3g

➢ Fiber: 12g

Servings: 4, Difficulty: Medium, Preparation Time: 60 minutes

CHAPTER EIGHT: Fatty Liver Dessert Recipes

1: Berry Chia Seed Pudding

Ingredients:

- 1/4 cup chia seeds
- 1 cup unsweetened almond milk (or any milk of choice)
- 1 tablespoon maple syrup or honey
- 1/2 teaspoon vanilla extract
- 1/2 cup mixed berries (such as strawberries, blueberries, raspberries)

Instructions:

1. In a mixing bowl, combine chia seeds, almond milk, maple syrup (or honey), and vanilla extract. Stir well to combine.
2. Let the mixture sit for 5 minutes, then stir again to prevent clumping. Cover and refrigerate for at least 2 hours or overnight until the mixture thickens.
3. Before serving, layer the chia seed pudding with mixed berries in serving glasses or bowls.
4. Optionally, garnish with additional berries or a drizzle of honey before serving.

Nutritional Value (per serving):

- ➢ Calories: 180 kcal
- ➢ Protein: 5g
- ➢ Carbohydrates: 23g
- ➢ Fat: 8g
- ➢ Fiber: 9g

Difficulty: Easy

Preparation Time: 5 minutes (+ refrigeration time)

2: Baked Apples with Cinnamon and Almonds

Ingredients:

- ➢ 2 large apples (such as Honeycrisp or Granny Smith)
- ➢ 2 tablespoons chopped almonds
- ➢ 1 tablespoon honey
- ➢ 1/2 teaspoon ground cinnamon
- ➢ 1/4 teaspoon ground nutmeg

Instructions:

- ➢ Preheat the oven to 375°F (190°C). Core the apples and cut them in half horizontally.
- ➢ In a small bowl, mix together chopped almonds, honey, cinnamon, and nutmeg.

- ➢ Fill each apple half with the almond mixture, pressing gently to pack it in.
- ➢ Place the filled apple halves on a baking sheet lined with parchment paper.
- ➢ Bake in the preheated oven for 20-25 minutes, or until the apples are tender and the topping is golden brown.
- ➢ Serve warm, optionally with a dollop of Greek yogurt or a sprinkle of additional cinnamon on top.

Nutritional Value (per serving):

- ➢ Calories: 180 kcal
- ➢ Protein: 3g
- ➢ Carbohydrates: 30g
- ➢ Fat: 6g
- ➢ Fiber: 6g

Difficulty: Easy

Preparation Time: 10 minutes

3: Mango Coconut Chia Pudding

Ingredients:

- ➢ 1/4 cup chia seeds
- ➢ 1 cup unsweetened coconut milk
- ➢ 1 tablespoon honey or maple syrup
- ➢ 1/2 teaspoon vanilla extract

➢ 1 ripe mango, diced

Instructions:

1. In a mixing bowl, combine chia seeds, coconut milk, honey (or maple syrup), and vanilla extract. Stir well to combine.

2. Let the mixture sit for 5 minutes, then stir again to prevent clumping. Cover and refrigerate for at least 2 hours or overnight until the mixture thickens.

3. Before serving, layer the chia seed pudding with diced mango in serving glasses or bowls.

4. Optionally, garnish with shredded coconut or a sprinkle of cinnamon before serving.

Nutritional Value (per serving):

➢ Calories: 220 kcal

➢ Protein: 5g

➢ Carbohydrates: 30g

➢ Fat: 10g

➢ Fiber: 9g

Difficulty: Easy

Preparation Time: 5 minutes (+ refrigeration time)

Ingredients:

- ➢ 2 ripe pears, halved and cored
- ➢ 2 tablespoons chopped walnuts
- ➢ 1 tablespoon honey
- ➢ 1/2 teaspoon ground cinnamon
- ➢ Pinch of ground cloves

Instructions:

1. Preheat the oven to 375°F (190°C). Place pear halves, cut side up, on a baking dish.
2. In a small bowl, mix together chopped walnuts, honey, cinnamon, and cloves.
3. Fill each pear half with the walnut mixture, pressing gently to pack it in.
4. Bake in the preheated oven for 20-25 minutes, or until the pears are tender and the topping is golden brown.
5. Serve warm, optionally with a dollop of Greek yogurt or a sprinkle of additional cinnamon on top.

Nutritional Value (per serving):

- ➢ Calories: 200 kcal
- ➢ Protein: 3g
- ➢ Carbohydrates: 30g

- ➤ Fat: 8g
- ➤ Fiber: 6g

Difficulty: Easy

Preparation Time: 10 minutes

5: Banana Almond Butter Bites

Ingredients:

- ➤ 2 ripe bananas, peeled and sliced into rounds
- ➤ 2 tablespoons almond butter (or any nut or seed butter of choice)
- ➤ 2 tablespoons unsweetened shredded coconut
- ➤ 1 tablespoon dark chocolate chips (optional)

Instructions:

1. Arrange the banana slices on a plate or baking sheet lined with parchment paper.
2. Spread almond butter onto half of the banana slices.
3. Top with the remaining banana slices to create sandwich bites.
4. Roll the edges of the banana bites in shredded coconut.
5. Optionally, sprinkle dark chocolate chips on top.
6. Place in the freezer for 30 minutes to firm up before serving.

Nutritional Value (per serving):

- ➤ Calories: 160 kcal

- ➢ Protein: 3g
- ➢ Carbohydrates: 20g
- ➢ Fat: 9g
- ➢ Fiber: 4g

Difficulty: Easy

Preparation Time: 10 minutes (+ chilling time)

6: Berry Yogurt Parfait with Granola

Ingredients:

- ➢ 1 cup Greek yogurt (or dairy-free yogurt alternative)
- ➢ 1/2 cup mixed berries (such as strawberries, blueberries, raspberries)
- ➢ 1/4 cup granola (choose a low-sugar option)
- ➢ 1 tablespoon honey or maple syrup (optional)

Instructions:

1. In a serving glass or bowl, layer Greek yogurt with mixed berries.
2. Sprinkle granola on top of the berries to add crunch and texture.
3. Optionally, drizzle honey or maple syrup over the parfait for added sweetness.
4. Serve immediately and enjoy!

Nutritional Value (per serving):

- ➢ Calories: 250 kcal
- ➢ Protein: 15g
- ➢ Carbohydrates: 30g
- ➢ Fat: 9g
- ➢ Fiber: 5g

Difficulty: Easy

Preparation Time: 5 minutes

7: Chocolate Avocado Mousse

Ingredients:

- ➢ 2 ripe avocados, peeled and pitted
- ➢ 1/4 cup unsweetened cocoa powder
- ➢ 1/4 cup maple syrup or honey
- ➢ 1 teaspoon vanilla extract
- ➢ Pinch of salt
- ➢ Fresh berries, for garnish (optional)

Instructions:

1. In a food processor or blender, combine the avocados, cocoa powder, maple syrup (or honey), vanilla extract, and salt.
2. Blend until smooth and creamy, scraping down the sides as needed to ensure thorough mixing.

3. Transfer the mousse to serving bowls or glasses.

4. Chill in the refrigerator for at least 30 minutes before serving.

5. Garnish with fresh berries before serving, if desired.

Nutritional Value (per serving):

➤ Calories: 200 kcal

➤ Protein: 3g

➤ Carbohydrates: 20g

➤ Fat: 14g

➤ Fiber: 7g

Difficulty: Easy

Preparation Time: 10 minutes (+ chilling time)

8: Cinnamon Baked Pear Crisp

Ingredients:

➤ 4 ripe pears, peeled, cored, and sliced

➤ 1 tablespoon lemon juice

➤ 1/4 cup rolled oats

➤ 2 tablespoons almond flour

➤ 1 tablespoon coconut oil, melted

➤ 1 tablespoon maple syrup or honey

➤ 1 teaspoon ground cinnamon

➤ Pinch of nutmeg

➤ Pinch of salt

Instructions:

1. Preheat the oven to 375°F (190°C). Lightly grease a baking dish.
2. In a bowl, toss the pear slices with lemon juice to prevent browning, then arrange them in the prepared baking dish.
3. In a separate bowl, combine the rolled oats, almond flour, melted coconut oil, maple syrup (or honey), cinnamon, nutmeg, and salt. Mix until well combined.
4. Sprinkle the oat mixture evenly over the pear slices in the baking dish.
5. Bake in the preheated oven for 25-30 minutes, or until the topping is golden brown and the pears are tender.
6. Allow to cool slightly before serving. Serve warm as is or with a dollop of Greek yogurt or coconut whipped cream, if desired.

Nutritional Value (per serving):

➢ Calories: 220 kcal
➢ Protein: 3g
➢ Carbohydrates: 40g
➢ Fat: 6g
➢ Fiber: 8g

Difficulty: Easy

Preparation Time: 15 minutes (+ baking time)

Ingredients:

- ➢ 4 medium apples, cored
- ➢ 2 tablespoons honey
- ➢ 1 teaspoon ground cinnamon
- ➢ 1/4 cup chopped walnuts
- ➢ 1/2 cup Greek yogurt (or dairy-free yogurt alternative)

Instructions:

1. Preheat the oven to 375°F (190°C).
2. In a small bowl, mix together honey, cinnamon, and chopped walnuts.
3. Place the cored apples in a baking dish and fill each apple cavity with the honey-cinnamon mixture.
4. Bake in the preheated oven for 25-30 minutes, or until the apples are tender.
5. Allow the baked apples to cool slightly before serving.
6. Serve each baked apple with a dollop of Greek yogurt on top.

Nutritional Value (per serving):

- Calories: 180 kcal
- Protein: 4g
- Carbohydrates: 30g
- Fat: 6g

- Fiber: 5g

Difficulty: Easy

Preparation Time: 10 minutes (+ baking time)

10: Mixed Berry Frozen Yogurt

Ingredients:

- 2 cups mixed berries (such as strawberries, blueberries, raspberries)
- 2 cups Greek yogurt (or dairy-free yogurt alternative)
- 2 tablespoons honey or maple syrup
- 1 teaspoon vanilla extract

Instructions:

1. Place the mixed berries, Greek yogurt, honey (or maple syrup), and vanilla extract in a blender or food processor.
2. Blend until smooth and creamy, scraping down the sides as needed to ensure thorough mixing.
3. Transfer the mixture to a shallow dish or ice cream maker.
4. If using a shallow dish, cover and freeze for 2-3 hours, stirring occasionally, until the mixture reaches a frozen yogurt consistency.

5. If using an ice cream maker, churn according to the manufacturer's instructions until the mixture reaches a soft serve consistency.

6. Serve the mixed berry frozen yogurt immediately as a soft serve or transfer to a container and freeze for an additional 1-2 hours for a firmer texture.

Nutritional Value (per serving):

- Calories: 150 kcal
- Protein: 10g
- Carbohydrates: 25g
- Fat: 1g
- Fiber: 5g

Difficulty: Easy

Preparation Time: 10 minutes (+ freezing time)

CONCLUSION

I want to express my sincere thanks for joining me on this journey through managing fatty liver disease. I hope the insights and recipes shared here have been helpful as you navigate this path towards better health.

As you move forward, remember that this journey is about patience, diligence, and self-care. By incorporating the tips and recipes from this book into your daily routine, I hope you find renewed energy and vitality.

Above all, I want you to feel empowered and hopeful. You have the ability to take control of your health and thrive despite the challenges you may face. Thank you for allowing me to be a part of your health journey, and I wish you all the best on your road to a healthier, happier life.